LUCKY DOG

LUCKY DOG

HOW BEING A VETERINARIAN
SAVED MY LIFE

DR. SARAH BOSTON

ANANSI

This edition published in 2014 by
House of Anansi Press Inc.
110 Spadina Avenue, Suite 801
Toronto, ON, M5V 2K4
Tel. 416-363-4343
Fax 416-363-1017
www.houseofanansi.com

Distributed in Canada by
HarperCollins Canada Ltd.
1995 Markham Road
Scarborough, ON, M1B 5M8
Toll free tel. 1-800-387-0117

Distributed in the United States by
Publishers Group West
1700 Fourth Street
Berkeley, CA 94710
Toll free tel. 1-800-788-3123

House of Anansi Press is committed to protecting our natural environment. As part of our efforts, the interior of this book is printed on paper that contains 100% post-consumer recycled fibres, is acid-free, and is processed chlorine-free.

18 17 16 15 14   1 2 3 4 5

Library and Archives Canada Cataloguing in Publication

Boston, Sarah, author
Lucky dog / Dr. Sarah Boston.

Issued in print and electronic formats.
ISBN: 978-1-77089-351-1 (pbk.). ISBN: 978-1-77089-352-8 (html).

1. Boston, Sarah, 1973–, Health. 2. Women veterinarians —
Biography. 3. Cancer—Patients—Biography. 4. Medical care.
I. Title.

SF613.B67A32014 636.089092 C2013907014-1
C2013-907015-X

Library of Congress Control Number: 2013918885

Cover design: Alysia Shewchuk
Text design and typesetting: Alysia Shewchuk

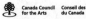

We acknowledge for their financial support of our publishing program the Canada Council for the Arts, the Ontario Arts Council, and the Government of Canada through the Canada Book Fund.

Printed and bound in Canada

MIX
Paper from
responsible sources
FSC® C004071
www.fsc.org

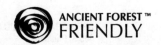

ANCIENT FOREST ™
FRIENDLY

For Stevie

CONTENTS

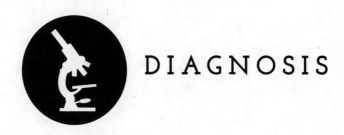

DIAGNOSIS

I WISH I WERE a dog. The lack of opposable thumbs part would be hard, and I do like talking a lot. I am also pathologically attached to my iPhone, but maybe there is an app that would allow me to continue to stay connected as a dog. The iPaw? Canine fashion has come a long way in the past few years, but I would miss shopping and dressing myself. I wouldn't miss the self-actualization and consciousness, but I would probably miss everyone recognizing my self-actualized consciousness. That would be hard. Even with having to give up the use of my hands, texting, the ability to speak, shopping, and the recognition of my full potential, I still wish that I were a dog today.

On Sunday night, six days ago, I was performing my nightly bedtime ritual, which involves washing my face with fantastically overpriced French cleanser and toner and then moisturizing with an equally overpriced French face cream. I believe this is worth it if the products can fulfill their promises of preventing the inescapable turkey neck that plagues women as they march into their late forties, the neck that seems to tarnish movie stars and human beings alike. No woman is immune and no amount of Botox or plastic surgery can erase the creping of the neck. It is the truth. Despite this, I am convinced that my routine is worth every penny and is working wonders. At thirty-seven and a half, I have the neck of a twenty-five-year-old. I alternate between extreme vanity and the suspicion that I may look like a cross between Ellen DeGeneres and Janice the Muppet. But back to vanity, I'm spreading on the cream, banishing forehead wrinkles, eye wrinkles, and smile lines. I move on to my the neck. Wait a second, what is that? I can feel a mass.

I do not say "bump" or "lump" or "swollen gland" because these fingers are trained fingers and I know instantly that it is a mass in my right thyroid gland. I know that it is new, and that it is not good. I'm away from home and staying with a dear friend in Calgary. I run into her bedroom and climb into bed with her. I ask her to feel my neck. She agrees that she can feel something and asks if it could be a swollen gland. She is not a doctor, but she plays one on TV (she is a health reporter). It is 11 p.m., and charged with this finding, but certain there is nothing that I can do about it right now, I retreat to my room. I try to reach my husband but I can't—his cellphone is dead. So I just lie awake all night thinking about what to do next.

The next morning, I get up early and try to see a doctor at a walk-in clinic, which is a mistake on many levels. In the waiting area, there is a guy wearing a SARS mask and a haggard woman with a bleeding gash on her head (and an inadequate piece of gauze taped to it), as well as a few other infectious-looking people. They all appear in more urgent need of attention than "neurotic veterinarian with self-diagnosed lump in her neck." The nurses are chatting away while people stand in line to be processed like cattle. I check in, but before I sit down, I ask how long the wait will be. The medical receptionist tells me that they are not permitted to give out wait times.

"Sure, I'm not going to hold you to it, but can you give me any idea? I have to call my office and I need to know what to tell them."

"We are not permitted to give out wait times."

"Okay, but can you tell me an average, like, will this be fifteen minutes or three hours?"

"I'm sorry, but we are not permitted to say."

Wow, thanks, superhelpful. I call work. I am doing a locum—a temporary position to fill in for another surgeon—at a private hospital in Calgary. It turns out that there is a patient waiting for me right now. We can't have that now, can we? I bail on the walk-in clinic. I am further delayed because I have to sign something that says I elected to leave against medical advice. What medical advice? Okay, whatever. This was a mistake. I sign it. I am going to be home in a week. I call my family doctor's office and get an appointment for Monday morning.

I arrive at work—a referral centre for animals. I am a veterinary surgeon with a subspecialty in surgical oncology (cancer surgery). I get through a couple of appointments, admitting one dog with an abdominal tumour that may need to be removed, along with the adjacent kidney. One of my colleagues is a veterinarian who is triple-boarded in three specialties: internal medicine, medical oncology, and radiation oncology—basically, this means he is a rock star to us vets, and a dog doctor to everyone else. I head to his office and ask him if he can feel my neck. I can see the instant recognition of a problem on his face and he says, "It's amazing what our fingers tell us sometimes." We sit and talk about what the mass could be: a cyst, hyperplasia (an increased production of normal cells), or a carcinoma (which is thyroid cancer), but mostly we talk about thyroid cancer because that is what we both think is going on. He tells me that the prognosis for most cases of thyroid carcinoma is good, especially in my age group. He tells me that I am pretty much the thyroid carcinoma poster girl and that I should go home.

So I fold on my locum early. I have never done anything like this in my life. Usually I drag myself into work, no matter what state my health is in, partly because I may be a workaholic and partly because I think the whole place would cease to function without me (see above, workaholic). I change my flight to leave on Wednesday and schedule an urgent appointment with my family doctor for Thursday. In this time, I am pretty sure the mass is growing.

Despite being a medical professional for nearly fifteen years, I have very few contacts in the human world. I reach for one: my colleague's brother, who is a head and neck surgeon in Toronto. After contacting him through his brother, I get a message back that he wants me to see an endrocrinologist for a workup before he sees me and he recommends one in Oakville. Great. I go to see my family doctor on Thursday as planned. Although I have given up

$2,500 in locum pay, my reputation, and a beautiful day of skiing in the Rockies with my friend Rob to make it back to see my doctor, he is not exactly on fire. I know what he is thinking. *She is a hypochondriac; she works with dog cancer all the time and automatically assumes that any symptom she has may be cancer related.* There's a possibility I have created some of this semi-hysterical-hypochondriac-woman image myself over the past two and a half years, since I go in and demand that any mole on my body that is even thinking of growing be excised immediately. When you deal with cancer every day, it is hard not to think the worst of lumps and bumps. I know that it is not always cancer, but I really do think I have cancer this time.

My doctor is about ten years younger than me. I try not to let this bother me, because I was a young doctor once, too. (I used to cringe when clients told me that I looked too young to be a veterinarian. Now it happens rarely, but I treasure this backwards compliment like I treasure getting ID'ed.) Despite his youth, my doctor has always been good to me.

I have treated well over a hundred dogs with thyroid carcinoma. I diagnose them, investigate if the cancer has spread, and perform the surgical removal. Just last week I submitted a paper that was a retrospective study of thyroid carcinoma in dogs (it will later be peer-reviewed and unanimously peer-rejected by several high-impact veterinary journals and sent to scientific paper purgatory, where it will die a slow and painful death). One of the findings from this now abandoned study was that early recognition and surgical intervention have a significant effect on prognosis. I get the feeling that my doctor has never diagnosed a case of thyroid cancer; he is spending too much time telling me how uncommon it is to be diagnosed with the disease. I think he is trying to soothe my anxiety, but his speech has the opposite effect. He feels my neck and my lymph nodes. He agrees that there is something there. Great. I thought that had been established. At least he agrees it's a thing. This appointment is just the beginning of our paradoxical relationship. He is the doctor but I know much more than he does about thyroid cancer. I have read the papers, I have seen the ultrasounds, and I have done the surgery. I am concerned.

He tells me that I have nothing to worry about, but that we will work it up "just in case." He sends me for blood work and an ultrasound and says he will call me if anything comes back "crazy." He tells me to try not to worry. I already know that nothing "crazy" will come back on the blood work, because with thyroid cancer, your thyroid levels can be normal, high, or low and they don't really suggest anything about the diagnosis or prognosis. So a necessary test to go through, yes, but not that helpful right now. At least I now have an official ultrasound requisition. I call the three locations I was given as options for my ultrasound and try to get the earliest appointment possible; I get one for a week later. I am told this is lucky and that I only got it because there has been a cancellation. I ask if they can do anything sooner; the receptionist says that if my doctor thinks it is urgent then yes, but otherwise no.

I am a pretty assertive woman (I think?) and I usually have no problem asking for what I want. But now I am wondering if I am assertive only when it is easy to be assertive and not when being assertive really matters, and that is, by definition, not assertive. I am not sure how I left my doctor's office without an urgent referral to a specialist in endocrinology. I try to tell myself that maybe it is because I am being a hypochondriac. I deal with cancer all the time so of course I think that it is cancer. It might be just a cyst. Maybe a cyst would get big this quickly. In four days, the mass has gone from something that I need to feel around for with my fingers to something that I can feel compressing my trachea and see in the mirror when I tilt my head to the side. It makes me cough occasionally and it is uncomfortable when I swallow. Trying to stay calm.

I go home. I am not relaxed. I happen to have access to a portable ultrasound machine because my husband, Steve, is a large animal veterinarian (more on that later). Given the fact that I cannot get an ultrasound appointment for another week, I decide that ultrasounding my own neck is the best course of action. Steve is reluctant to give me this piece of equipment because it is not a good idea for vets to treat people or for any type of doctor to diagnose or treat themselves. But I beg him to bring his ultrasound machine home. My main motivation in this bizarre exercise is to find a big cyst, laugh about how crazy I acted, calm down, and just wait out the glacial pace of our socialized Canadian health care system with the knowledge that my mass is very likely benign. Cysts are easy to diagnose on ultrasound because they are full of fluid, and this looks very different from any other type of tissue.

I am alone in the kitchen. The lights are off. I start evaluating the mass with the probe. I find it easily, since it's huge. Then I orient myself on the screen: I can see my carotid artery; there's my larynx; there is my trachea; and there is the normal thyroid tissue around the mass. I investigate the 3- to 4-centimetre mass within my right thyroid gland. It is definitely not cystic because there is very little fluid. It is solid tissue and the tissue is distinct from the thyroid gland itself. I recognize that I could be jumping to conclusions because of my vocation, and that it is actually pretty messed up to ultrasound your own thyroid mass and then to interpret the images yourself, but it looks like cancer to me and I know what I know. I also find a small nodule on the left side. It is only 1 centimetre and it looks benign to me. This exercise did nothing to help calm me down. Still trying not to worry.

Another sleepless night follows. It is filled with some Internet research on the endrocinologist who was recommended to me; an ethical debate with myself about whether or not I could forge an online referral from my doctor (because I have his physician number on the ultrasound requisition); a brief but fruitless search for private clinics in Canada (they exist, but only to take care of the specific health needs of rich businessmen, it seems); a short-lived and frightening search for endrocrinologists in Buffalo; downloading articles on thyroid carcinoma from PubMed; and writing a few dark and bizarre emails to close friends. I have already read a lot of papers on thyroid carcinoma in humans and dogs, but I start reading specific articles on distinguishing between benign and malignant thyroid masses using ultrasound. There is not one characteristic that can diagnose a thyroid carcinoma on ultrasound (you need a biopsy for that), but there are several criteria on ultrasound that are very suggestive of cancer, and my thyroid mass seems to fulfill most of them. My covert self-ultrasound has led to a covert self-diagnosis of thyroid cancer.

The next morning at 8 a.m., I head back to my doctor's office armed with my husband (whom I have asked not to let me leave without an urgent referral to a specialist), a USB key that contains images of my thyroid mass, and lots of tears (real ones, not just for dramatic effect). My doctor is gracious and sees me right away. I explain to him that I think the mass is getting bigger and that I ultrasounded it with a colleague last night (a.k.a. my husband, who was actually hiding from the madness in the living room). I proceed to relay my alarming findings to him with a verbal report (despite lacking the official title of radiologist).

"There is a 3.5-centimetre mass within the right thyroid gland that is hypoechoic compared to the thyroid tissue, with mixed echogenicity, including areas of mineralization. It is taller than it is wide. I can see a large blood vessel running through the middle of it. There is a small cystic area as well. Based on what I have read, these findings fulfill most of the ultrasonographic criteria of malignancy and I want an urgent referral to an endocrinologist. I am concerned."

I hand him the USB key and ask him if he would like to look at it with me. He says that is probably not necessary because I obviously still need an ultrasound with a radiologist. I realize that it is likely my doctor has never seen an ultrasound of a thyroid gland, except perhaps in medical school, so looking at these images will be somewhat meaningless. Human general practitioners (GPs) do not have the luxury of following their patients through their diagnostic tests, like I do. In my world, I can watch the ultrasound, go over the CT scan with the radiologist, take the patient to surgery, and look at the histopathology (a microscopic examination of the tissue by a pathologist) with the pathologist. In my GP's world, imaging, biopsies, and blood work are reduced to a black-and-white report with a bottom line from a pathologist or radiologist. The initial doctor will never get a sense of what the mass looks like.

The strange paradox in our relationship continues. Normally, your doctor tells you that you have cancer, not the other way around. I have to get him to come to terms with my cancer and accept it so that we can move forward and he can get me an urgent referral. He has all the power. He agrees that I need an immediate biopsy. I am not sure if this is because he thinks I will be in a loony bin if that does not happen urgently (possibly true) or because he believes my superb ultrasound report, but I don't actually care. He says he would like to send me to a head and neck surgeon in Guelph who can do a biopsy and that he will do an urgent referral. It is Friday, so this will likely happen next week. He also says he will try to move up the ultrasound appointment so that it will be done before the surgeon sees me. He says I am still going to have to wait it out at least over the weekend but that his nurse will call me later today with a plan. I ask him off-the-cuff if he would send me home with some Valium and he immediately writes me a script for Ativan. What the hell. I fill it. I need sleep.

I spend the day trying to be calm. I do yoga. I get a pedicure. I go shoe shopping and find some perfect, insanely expensive boots that I don't need. Sometimes I struggle to differentiate between my wants and needs. I also struggle with the difference between reality and make-believe at times, which is why I can never go to Disney World. I justify the purchase, deciding that if the mass is benign, the boots will celebrate life with my benign thyroid mass, and if the mass is cancer, then there is no need to save money for the future and I deserve some kick-ass boots. I've always thought that if I knew how long I was going to live, it would really help with my shoe budget.

At 2:30, mid–shoe purchase, the nurse from my doctor's office calls to tell me that the head and neck surgeon they wanted to send me to is on holidays and that my ultrasound appointment cannot be moved up. Luckily, I am still riding my boot-purchase-induced serotonin high. I ask her who else they can refer me to and she is stumped. She says I can ask the surgeon in Toronto if he can see me, but they really don't have a lot of "pull" to get patients help in Toronto. I tell her that I have no pull because most of the specialists need the referring doctor to say it is urgent. I ask her to refer me to the endrocrinologist I originally wanted to go to. She asks me if I know the number; somehow I actually remember it. I tell her how to find the web site and that the online referral process is quite straightforward.

I phone the endocrinologist's office a bit later to check in. My doctor's office has not sent in the referral yet. I ask the receptionist I am speaking to if she has a minute and tell her the peculiar tale of the dog-cancer surgeon with the mass in her neck. I have her attention.

"How's Thursday?"

"Really? Thank you, that would be great." I could cry.

I contact my doctor's office again. I tell them I have my appointment and I just need them to send over the referral letter. And now I have to wait. Only six days, but it is going to be hard—and it is only the first step toward getting a diagnosis and treatment.

I compare my experience with my patients'. The dogs I treat for thyroid carcinoma come in for their appointment in the morning and have thoracic radiographs (chest X-rays), blood work, and an ultrasound of their neck all done on the same day. Depending on the results, we may do a needle biopsy of their neck mass that day as well, and will get the report back from the pathologist later that afternoon. From there, we schedule a CT and surgery for the next day. The surgery takes me approximately thirty minutes or less. I love doing thyroidectomies (removing one of the paired thyroid glands)—they are fun and quick. I call it a "neck neuter" because the mass looks like a testicle as it is being removed. The mass is submitted for histopathology and the preliminary results are available within twenty-four hours. The dogs recover in the intensive care unit (ICU) and go home the following day. In ten to fourteen days they will return for suture removal and an appointment with a medical oncologist to discuss the histopathology results and whether or not we recommend chemotherapy. Chemotherapy can start the same day.

And that is why I wish I were a dog. Because I would take better care of me.

I have clients who tell me this all the time. They say that if they get sick, they want to check themselves in to our animal hospital, because the care is so much better, so much faster, and we care so much more. It's a joke. Sort of. I will spend the next year dividing my time between having and treating cancer, between being the doctor and being the patient. It is a perspective I would never have asked for, and I don't mean to be critical but, well, I just can't help myself. I'm a little critical of the human system. We need to do better. We need to care more. We need to advocate more. We need to cherish ourselves the way we do our most perfect companions—our dogs.

BEFORE I TELL YOU more about my thyroid situation, I should tell you a little about myself. I am a veterinary surgical oncologist, but more simply, I am a small animal veterinarian. I think most children decide that they are going to become a veterinarian at some point. Sometimes they don't know what it means, but becoming an animal saver or a pet-erinarian (so cute!) sounds like a great gig. When people find out that I am a veterinarian, they usually ask me when I decided on that career path. I tell them I have wanted to be a veterinarian since I was six. This isn't technically true, but I did write it down at school when I was six, and it's the earliest documentation available that I wanted to help animals for a living. I can't remember ever deciding to be a vet; it was just something I had always known. This is a feeling a lot of us in the profession share. It is part of our fabric to love and understand animals and want to help them.

I don't think that I had an epiphany or an aha moment about my career choice. Maybe I just can't remember it. I was recently at an outdoor brewpub with my dog and a bunch of vets and vet students. A two-year-old who was there with her young parents came screeching up to us. She was having trouble containing her excitement about seeing the dog, and shrieks of enthusiasm were bubbling out of her as she approached. She was fearless. The toddler was trying to have a conversation with my dog; she got her face as close as she could to his face so she could look him right in the eyes, which meant she was down on her hands and knees. The two of them were engaged in non-verbal communication in a way that those of us with speech at our disposal simply can't replicate. Her dad came over to retrieve her. I told him that she was hanging out with a bunch of vets and was one of us. I think this is why I can't remember when I decided to become a vet. I was probably too young to speak to people and too busy having a serious conversation with a dog about it.

I decided to go back to my roots to try to figure this out. I interviewed my family to ask them when I decided to become a vet. I started with my dad.

"Dad, when did I decide to become a veterinarian?"

This gave my dad the opportunity to do what he usually does—use the question to give one of his favourite pieces of advice or to tell his favourite story, or both, possibly summing up his main thesis with one of the thousand literary quotes he has at his disposal. He may or may not answer the actual question.

"I was always very supportive of you becoming a veterinarian. Do you want to know why?" (He does not wait for me to answer.) "Because being a veterinarian is a vocational ticket. That's why. Nobody can ever take that away from you."

Okay, that was the advice part. The importance of having a vocational ticket is a concept I was brainwashed with from an early age. Going to university was not enough. You needed to be a something—a lawyer, a teacher, a veterinarian, a doctor, or another type of professional— because no one can take that away from you and you will always have a job. I can't become a writer because someone might try to take that away from me. Here comes the semi-related story from my dad.

"When you were eight, we used to drive to Banff to take Nutmeg for her obedience training."

Nutmeg was not my family's first dog, but she was my first dog. She was a golden retriever who was supposed to be for the whole family, and she was, but she was mine. She picked me. She slept beside my bed, comforted me when I was sad, played with me, and I walked her all the time. I understood everything that she never said to me. When I came home from school, she would find her favourite toy, or anything that would fit in her mouth (having something in her mouth was an essential part of the display), and make a crazy squeaking noise and smile so hard that her ears would stick out to the sides. This production would go on for about ten minutes. It was pure joy. My translation of this spectacle: "You're home! Where were you? I love you! I'm so happy to see you! I missed you! Look at my toy!"

My family decided that I was going to be the one to train Nutmeg. Nutmeg and I took it seriously and we

practised all the time. It might have been our intense bond, or the fact that I was an exceptional and gifted animal trainer, or the fact that my parents are a tad competitive when it comes to their kids, or just that golden retrievers are incredibly trainable, but whatever it was, it was canine training magic. We rocked the obedience ring. My dad took me every week.

"During the final class," he continued, "we had the graduation competition. In the end, it was down to you and Nutmeg and the middle-aged German and his husky. You had to do the final long sit-stay to see who was going to break the tie. The husky cracked under the pressure and broke his stay, so when the final points were tallied up, you won! We won! You and Nutmeg were top of the class! I can still see the German saying 'Congratulations' to you through his gritted teeth and forced grimace, and how much he hated losing to a little girl and her golden retriever. And I remember thinking: Well, sir, we beat you in two world wars, and tonight...we beat you *again*!"

My dad is having trouble getting this last part out because he is laughing so hard. I inherited the ability to crack myself up from him. Not everyone finds me as funny as I do, but I can't help it if some people are obtuse. I kill me. Also, I would like to apologize to any Germans out there who find this part offensive. My dad is very British and quite old.

So maybe this was the defining moment? The ride home with my gloating father and Nutmeg, holding a puppy Heisman Trophy on my lap and enjoying the sweet smell of victory and the rush of competition? Maybe it was also the realization that even though beating the husky and the

German seemed impossible—maybe it was their matching ice-blue eyes and northern intensity—I was still able to triumph over German efficiency through hard work and by being a total geek. I'm not sure. I needed to do more research.

So I asked my mom, "When did I decide to become a veterinarian?"

"Do you want me to write this part of the book for you?"

"No, Mom, I want to write it myself, but I need information."

"Well, you were very young and *very* advanced. We took you down to the local veterinary clinic in Canmore, and you started to volunteer there when you were just eight years old."

Obviously eight was a big year for me. I think I might have peaked too early. Looking back, it is a bit ridiculous that I was an eight-year-old volunteer—something you could only get away with in a small town in the eighties. But I was fascinated by the local veterinary clinic and spent all of my weekends and holidays there. I was eager to do anything to help. Mopping the floor made me happy, and I would follow the veterinary technicians around and do anything they asked me. During this time, veterinarians were even more frugal than they are now. We used to spend time cleaning and resterilizing syringes. Although you could argue that this is quite environmentally conscious, it is also insane. To pay technicians their hourly wage to clean out plastic syringes—which cost pennies and are only supposed to be used once and are impossible to clean properly—in order to package and sterilize them in an autoclave, which also costs money to run, is in

the dictionary under *false economy*. I didn't know this at the time; I just focused on flushing the blood clots out of the syringes like it was all that I lived for. I cleaned exam rooms, walked dogs, counted pills, cleaned cages, played with the clinic cats, took out the garbage, and answered the phone. By the time I was ten, I was allowed to go to the clinic *by myself* to take care of boarding patients on the weekend and was allowed to drop off the daily deposit at the bank on the way home on my ten-speed. Again, small town, very advanced child, the eighties.

The best part was when I got to watch surgery: mostly spays and neuters, but sometimes surgically draining cat abscesses, which might actually have been a defining moment, because I have not met a veterinarian who does not derive a perverse delight from lancing a big, stinky abscess in any species. It's cathartic. At the end of my second summer there, Cara, the veterinarian I volunteered for, gave me $150 to thank me for all of my hard work. It was a cheque from the head office in Calgary, so it meant that they had said it was okay to pay me, too. One hundred and fifty big ones! I had no idea I could make so much money helping animals. Find your passion and the dollars will start to roll in. (The truth is, veterinary medicine is not a lucrative profession, despite what people may think.)

"That reminds me," my mom started, "have you talked to Cara lately?"

"No, Mom, not since I told her that I graduated from vet school in 1996."

"I think you should reach out to her. I am sure she would like to know how you are doing."

"Okay, I will get in touch."

"You used to come home from volunteering and over dinner you would tell us about all of the surgeries you watched that day and it would make us all sick to our stomachs, but you loved it. You always loved surgery."

Then my mom launches into her favourite imitation of me at the dinner table telling my family about the surgeries I'd seen that day, and she does this funny accent that is supposed to be me as a child, saying, "Guess what I saw today, Mummy?" but she sounds more like Oliver, the British orphan from the musical *Oliver!* than my child self. And I have never said "Mummy" in my life. I pretty much came out of the womb saying "Mom."

It's true though; I did love watching surgery. It was my reward for all the hard work I did. I would help get the cats ready by shaving and cleaning their bellies before they were spayed. One of the more abrasive technicians, who was not particularly fond of me or of having a very advanced eight-year-old take over her job responsibilities, would yell, "Watch her tit! Watch her TIT!" at me when she thought that I was shaving a little too vigorously around a cat's nipple. I am still traumatized by this and cannot shave a cat's abdomen to this day without her words burning in my brain. It had not occurred to me until then that cats had tits, or that they had so many of them. For the record, her tits were just fine—all of them. I was very careful with the cat's tits.

During surgery, I would sit on a wooden stool in the corner watching and asking questions. It was there that I came to the alarming realization that when you eat an animal, you are eating its muscle, and that dog and cat muscles look the same as meat. It took a few more years

for me to stop eating meat, but I put this all together when I was around fourteen years old. I stopped wearing leather for years as well, but now I am a big fat hypocrite because vegetarian shoes are simply horrific looking.

I continued my investigation with my brother, asking him when I decided to become a veterinarian.

"I don't know. You always wanted to be a veterinarian."

My brother has known me for a long time. Pretty much from day one.

"All I remember is the time you brought that fetal pig home after Mom and Dad moved to Ottawa and you put it in the fridge without telling me. I was hungry and thought it was food, so I got it out of the wrapper and then realized it was a fetal pig!" My brother says this incredulously, as if it could not have been more shocking to pull back the tinfoil to reveal a severed human head. "After that I wasn't hungry any more."

That was a bit of a dark chapter in our relationship. We were living in Saskatoon, Saskatchewan, at the time. I was going into grade twelve and my brother was going into his first year of university. My parents were planning to move to Ottawa and were entertaining the idea that my brother and I stay in Saskatchewan and live together in a student condo. My brother wanted to stay in Saskatoon because he hates change. I wanted to stay in Saskatoon for a number of reasons:

1. We had moved to Saskatoon from Canmore, Alberta, three years earlier and I was only just starting to recover from my total teen meltdown caused by the trauma of moving.

2. My parents were only able to persuade me to leave Canmore in the first place by telling me that Saskatoon had the only vet school in western Canada. I reluctantly agreed to go with them and not get my own apartment at the age of thirteen.

3. I had just been voted senior pin at my high school, which is like being class president. How could I leave when the whole school was counting on me to lead?

4. As I like to tell people, I was very popular in high school, but not in a *Mean Girls* bitchy way, like you are thinking. I was a friend to all; from nerd to skid to prep to band kids, I brought people together. Once, during a spare, I walked to the store with some skids who were skipping class; the mission was to get smokes (them) and candy (me). I held back one skid's hair while she puked up neon-green slime in the alley four times. She then lit a smoke and I went back to class. I was a social chameleon.

5. I was concerned I might not be popular in a new high school because my leadership skills, social adaptability, and wit might not be as apparent to people in Ontario, which would be tragic.

6. My parents were not moving to a city in Ontario with a vet school.

7. Ontario had grade thirteen at the time, which meant five years of high school instead of four. I did not

skip kindergarten and start grade one at the tender
age of five because of my advanced skills in reading
and napping only to have that year stolen away from
me by the Ontario government.

8. I had my driver's licence now and was planning on
getting two kittens, which means I had everything I
needed to live without parents.

So my brother and I stayed behind and lived together in
Saskatoon. We had some skills, but not the full complement
required for running a household. I also decided that getting two kittens and rescuing a psychologically damaged
shelter puppy that was almost impossible to house-train
(see later, Gilligan) would be a fine idea for our new living
situation, sans parents. For me, living in a house without
animals was like living in a house without furniture.

Back to the pig story: to teach us about anatomy, my
grade twelve biology teacher handed out formaldehyde-
soaked fetal pigs for us to dissect. He told us we had to
keep them cool and that we would only get one piglet each.
We had to care for our piglets like the pretend baby they
give to teenaged girls in "life-skills" classes to show them
how much work it is to take care of a real baby. Somehow,
this exercise always made a baby seem more like a cute
accessory than a life-destroying disaster. My fetal pig was
fortunately not holding me back or making me consider
the darker aspects of teen pregnancy.

There was no proper adult in the house to tell me that
I was not allowed to keep my formaldehyde-soaked fetal
pig in the refrigerator. As I remember, my biology teacher

"encouraged" us to store them in a cool place (e.g., a fridge) and I feel that he was complicit in this bad decision. On further reflection, leaving a formaldehyde-soaked fetal pig adjacent to your food is not something I would recommend, or even suggest, like my teacher did. Formaldehyde is toxic. Luckily, I did not become pregnant in high school during my fetal pig project, since formaldehyde debatably causes birth defects and maybe cancer, too.

So I guess it's possible I gave myself cancer from my improper embalmed-fetal-pig storage. It's a textbook case of latent formaldehyde-induced thyroid cancer. I am not sure why I did not just leave my piglet outside. I lived in Saskatchewan. Saskatchewan is like a freezer 80 percent of the time, like a fridge 19 percent of the time, and warm 1 percent of the time. My piglet would have been fine outside, but I felt insecure about leaving it out there for fear that someone might take it or wild animals might get into it, causing me to be deemed a bad student and not at all ready for parenthood because I couldn't even keep track of my unborn pig.

My attachment to my fetal pig was also due to strong visions of my failed grade six mealworm science project. Our teacher instructed us to bring home a jar of mealworms and watch their life cycle. My dad refused to allow them in the house, no doubt worried that they might escape and result in a mealworm infestation, so I put them near the heater in the garage to keep them warm. The next morning, I discovered I had accidently delivered them all to a toasty death. I didn't have time to breed more mealworms for my mealworm project and I learned nothing about mealworm breeding and genetics.

Not this time, I said. Not this time.

After my fetal pig project ended, the refrigerator became a food-friendly place again. My journey with science, and eventually veterinary medicine, continued; my brother's distaste for biology confirmed, he followed a career in philospophy (yes, I said career in philosophy). Following several other incidents involving the neurotic untrained pound puppy and the cats, and arguments over who was supposed to help care for them and clean up their messes, we went our separate ways. As is the case for most adult brothers and sisters, we have become closer now that the forced-togetherness phase of our lives is over.

Next stop on my exploration of being a veterinarian is my husband, Steve.

"Why did I decide to become a veterinarian?"

"You were already a veterinarian when I met you."

"But I had been one for only a few months. Can you speculate?"

"You became a veterinarian because animals are your passion."

"I think that's true. Why did you become a veterinarian?"

"You know why."

"I know, but I am doing my research."

"Well, my first degree was in math and statistics. I was going to be an actuary, but then I realized it would be a boring, awful job for me. I grew up working with stan- dardbred horses on my grandparents' farm, so that is why I decided to become a vet. I wanted to work with animals and I wanted to work outside."

The thought of Steve being trapped in an office every day, calculating the statistical probability of death, dismemberment, and disaster for an insurance company, is hilarious. Maybe you have to know him to think it is funny. Imagine a modern-day James Herriot putting on a suit and tie and heading to work to calculate the financial consequences of risk. It makes no sense. Sometimes it just takes the courage to follow your dreams. Steve is now a large animal veterinarian, which means he takes care of cows and horses (not that he is large, or that the animals he works on are overly large, like elephants or giraffes).

We met when I was an intern and he was a senior veterinary student in Guelph, Ontario. This might sound scandalous or interesting but it wasn't, especially now that we've been together for seventeen years. It might also sound unique—veterinary couple—but it is actually pretty common and even a bit clichéd in our circle. We are birds of a feather; we flock together. I had explicit plans to marry a lawyer or a famous artist and live in a very fancy loft with a lot of art and money. Then I met Steve, a soon-to-be large animal veterinarian with very blue eyes and the ability to make me blush when he looked at me and, well, that was that.

People always ask us if we are going to open a practice together, because we are both vets and they think this would be the ultimate goal of the unique veterinary couple. Sorry to burst your bubble, people—the answer is no. We can't own a practice together because Steve works on cows and horses and I work on dogs and cats. He works on getting large animals pregnant and helping them to get up when they go down, and I am a specialist, removing tumours in small animals. Unfortunately, there is just no overlap here; the practice model is inherently flawed.

It is great to be married to a veterinarian, even if our jobs are very different, because veterinarians have so many commonalities: our love of animals, for one, and the disappointment we share when we discover that not everyone loves animals the way we do or cares for them the way that they should. There is also a mutual understanding that sometimes things can go sideways at work and that time can get the better of us. Steve and I can both recognize the pressure our clients put on us, which is only topped by the pressure we put on ourselves; we share a desire for perfectionism and a tendency toward extreme disappointment in ourselves when things do not go perfectly. It's nice to come home to someone who can truly appreciate what my day has been like and can relate, without having to explain too much.

Nutmeg is long gone, so I can't ask her why I became a veterinarian, but if I could, I think she would say, "It was me. It was because of me."

She has a point. It was definitely her.

I'M SURE YOU SPENT the whole last chapter wondering what has been going on with this neck lump. Well, don't worry, you have not missed a thing. I had hoped that by now I could be telling a great story about how the mind can play tricks on you when you are a veterinary surgical oncologist with a lump; that really it was just my imagination running away with me for that crazy week. But it has now been five weeks since I found a mass in my neck, freaked out, ultrasounded myself, and ambushed my general practitioner into a referral to an endocrinologist. Five weeks in which very little has happened.

So, five weeks ago I met with my GP, and I will admit it was not my best week. I got very little sleep and the sleep I did have was sponsored by my new best friend, Ativan. The combination of the lack of sleep, Ativan hangover, and stress resulted in some serious lapses in memory and judgement. Retrospectively, driving and working may not have been advisable, but I plowed through.

Everyone had great advice for me, like "Just try to keep your mind off it by focusing on your work"; hard to do, especially when my work is diagnosing and treating cancer in dogs and cats. A few days after meeting with my GP, I had an internal consultation for a colleague on a case of a dog with thyroid cancer and had to watch the CT come up, slice by slice, with gross evidence of the spread of the cancer to the lungs and lymph nodes. I panicked, thinking that this was what would happen to me if I ever managed to see a specialist and get a CT scan done. This dog had widespread metastasis, so surgical removal of the thyroid gland was unlikely to be helpful. I turned to my colleague. "Sorry, this case is not surgical. There is nothing I can do."

"Try yoga and deep relaxation," a few friends advised. So I went to yoga, where I watched the mass pop out of my neck in the mirror as I stretched, balanced, and took deep breaths.

I heard the obligatory "Get lots of rest and eat well," but every time I ate something, I felt the mass when I swallowed. I tried to sleep, but I couldn't because it was uncomfortable. My mass is always there, as ever-present on my mind as it is pushing on my neck.

Four weeks ago, I met the endocrinologist for the first time. He was lovely, and after giving me a light spanking (metaphorically speaking) for ultrasounding my own neck, he assured me that I do not have cancer. And I believed him (sort of). It calmed me down to hear him say, "You don't have cancer," as he patted my knee. It brought me to tears. My GP told me the same thing, but that brought me to tears in a different way—it made me more certain that he had no idea what he was talking about, and that I was surely on the brink of death from my abnormally aggressive, widely metastatic, neck-eating thyroid cancer.

But the lovely endocrinologist started wielding his telephone and making things happen. *Boom*, ultrasound that afternoon. *Boom*, talked to a colleague and secured the promise of an ultrasound-guided biopsy the next week! Then he told me a story about another patient of his—a pregnant woman who had a thyroid mass like mine. He apparently also told her that she did not have cancer. He gave her the option to have a biopsy if she wanted but told her it was nothing to worry about. She felt better, just like I did, and planned to wait until after she had the baby to have a biopsy done. But for some reason her husband pushed her to get the biopsy done sooner, so she did. It turns out that she had a thyroid carcinoma that had metastasized to her lymph nodes. This was a very interesting narrative, but I am not sure what I was supposed to learn from it. Was he trying to tell me not to trust him, or that everyone needs an advocate to navigate their way through the health care system? Maybe it was both. Either way, I wanted the biopsy.

I marvelled at his ability to assess me. Not just the mass, but all of me. He sized me up quickly: career woman; works in veterinary oncology; enough knowledge to be dangerous and/or a pain in the ass; no children and acts like she is twenty-seven, despite being thirty-seven; wants neck mass out yesterday; does not want to wait in line; is not patient.

I size up my clients in a similar fashion: mid-forties woman; single; pleasant but very stressed; teary-eyed;

wearing polycotton-blend sweatshirt airbrushed with the image of a dog of the same breed as hers that she likes to wear to the vet's office and other dog-related events; does agility/showing/breeding/field trialing with this dog, who happens to be a world champion of agility/showing/breeding/field trialing. This dog is not a part of her life. This dog *is* her life, her companion, her hobby, and her joy. Dog equals life companion.

Next one: gay couple, one of whom is immaculately dressed in a suit and has a very fancy job and a very fancy income. The dog is a very fancy breed. Maybe a Wegman-esque Weimaraner or a chocolate lab. The one in the suit is a bit more demanding, agitated, and easily frustrated. My inner gay man is just as bitchy as he is, and I know that it is just the stress talking anyway, so it doesn't bother me. The other half of the couple is softer, wears a plaid flannel shirt and cords, and is beside himself with worry and grief and cries intermittently during the appointment. Dog equals child substitute.

Next one I know well because it was me: early thirties; single woman; attractive and/or thinks she is attractive and/or works really hard on being attractive; high-powered job; was in university for a long time. Dog is big, usually male, and has been with her through various degrees, boyfriends, twentysomething dramas, and moves. Her dog has always been there for her during her busy times, as a willing companion and protector for study breaks, walks, runs, coffee dates, movie nights, and shopping when other friends were not available on short notice. She cries, then apologizes for crying and tries to pull herself together, plays with her cellphone, then cries again, apologizes, and says, "I am not usually like this; it is just *this* dog." High alert: this dog is her soulmate.

Right after my appointment, my endocrinologist had another doctor call me to arrange a needle biopsy, as promised. My endocrinologist asked that they get me in quickly for the biopsy because I am a "colleague," which was sweet—or patronizing—it is hard to tell sometimes with physicians. The biopsy doctor told me that he couldn't do it for twelve days. He let me know that he would have to work through his lunch hour to squeeze me in, but not for twelve days.

Around three weeks ago, absolutely nothing had happened.

I had my ultrasound-guided biopsy done a little over two weeks ago. The specialist who did my biopsy was the third doctor to tell me that he thought the mass was probably benign. He proceeded to tell me that the cytology test I was having done is not a very accurate way of distinguishing between a benign or malignant thyroid tumour. In order to find out what kind of tumour it is, I needed to have it surgically removed and have histopathology done. I knew all this, of course.

"So why are you not just having surgery if you are so worried?" he asked. Great question.

I tried not to lose it. I told him that I was aware of all the facts and that having it removed ASAP would be my first choice, but I was not in charge and I needed to get this test done before I could even see the surgeon.

He started the test by ultrasounding my neck to evaluate the mass. He used the images on the ultrasound to watch the biopsy needle and guide it as it entered the mass, and he took a sample by aspirating, or putting suction on the needle with a syringe. We could see that there were actually two masses: the biggie on the right side that was causing all the fuss, and a 1-centimetre mass on the left side that looked very well-behaved. I was not worried about the small mass—I'd seen it on my self-ultrasound— but he wanted to biopsy both of them while he was there. Perfect. Now we'll have two pointless equivocal test results that are difficult to interpret and require surgery and histopathology for a definitive diagnosis. He stabbed away at my neck with the needle, right beside my larynx and trachea. He told me that I could absolutely not swallow, move, or talk (or else I would risk him lacerating my trachea or possibly my carotid artery, which is also right there). Right, I got it, didn't move. It hurt—a lot.

While I was having this done, I thought about all of the brave, non-complaining dogs that have been in my hands for this exact test, and I silently promised my future patients not to do any more thyroid aspirations on them without sedation and pain medication. We punish the good dogs, the ones that just lie still, trusting us and our restraint, tails thumping on the table as we stab them in the neck with the needle. The dogs who resist are the "bad" dogs, the fractious ones that need sedation. If I were a dog right now, I would definitely be a bad dog. I wished I had been sedated; it would make it so much easier.

It has now been one week since I received the call from the lovely endocrinologist, who was really so lovely. He had some lovely and benevolent news that the cytology report on the thyroid mass had come back as benign. "But we knew that," he said, chuckling. I felt relieved, but I still couldn't completely let go of the stress and the feeling that I wanted this mass out. I was over being patronized and told that I was just acting like a hypochondriac because I knew too much about cancer. It's true, I know stuff. I know that cytology is not the best tool to differentiate between benign and malignant thyroid disease. I know that 85 percent of thyroid masses or nodules in women are benign. I also know that if a mass is over 2 centimetres (mine is now 3.8 centimetres) malignancy is more likely, so the best plan is to remove it. I also know that it doesn't matter how many times someone tells me it is probably benign, or even that the cytology is benign, I will think that this is cancer until the mass is out, in a jar of formalin, and I have a histopathology report in my hands that says otherwise.

In five weeks, all I really got was two ultrasounds (three if you include mine), an ultrasound-guided needle biopsy for a cytology test that is unreliable, and three doctors (GP, endocrinologist, and the biopsy doctor) telling me that I don't have cancer.

My lovely endocrinlogist finally refers me to the surgeon, who is my colleague's brother. I still have to wait another week for an appointment with the surgeon and it sounds like surgery won't be for another four to six weeks after that. All of this is a lesson in how to torment a surgical oncologist: give her a mass in her neck and make her wait.

ALL THE WAITING IS hard, whether it is you, a friend, a family member, or your dog who has cancer. A lot of dog owners feel the need to take some control of their dog's fate, and that leads them to the Internet and, often, that leads them to me. In some ways, I guess it is flattering to be someone whom people find on the Internet when searching for cancer treatment for their pet. Flattering in a creepy, cyberstalking kind of way. Our human counterparts have walls for this. Their email addresses aren't out there, and if they are, they have people to answer emails on their behalf. You will not have an online chat with a specialist of your choice about your own health problems. But your dog is different. Veterinary specialists are different, especially those of us working at a university. We are in the public domain.

I can always feel the sadness overwhelming these pet owners, even in the boldest and most demanding of emails. While this direct contact can be a bit intrusive, and my professional self knows that I should just pass the email off on someone else to book them an appointment, I don't. I know that they are at home, looking at their beloved dog with cancer, trying to find hope. They are wondering if anyone is ever going to love them as much as their dog. Unconditional love is a basic human need, and so often it is non-humans that fulfill it. Hope can be taken away from someone so easily: a bad diagnosis, a comment from a well-meaning or not-so-well-meaning acquaintance, a veterinarian who doesn't think dogs should have aggressive cancer treatment, or bad economic times can all drain us of hope. When a human family member has cancer, people usually come together. Everyone is fighting on the same team. When a family pet has cancer, it is polarizing and isolating. People break into their strong opinion–, weak data–based camps about the ethics, finances, and benefits of treating cancer in pets that they have never met.

So I always cave and email people back. Maybe it's a codependency or ego thing. It doesn't take too much time, just a quick email to tell them that we are happy to meet with them to assess their dog and go over all of the options. I try to comfort them with the knowledge that there are *always* options. Hope can be extinguished quickly, but you can give it back quickly, too. And that is how I met Carney.

Subject: my dog with bone cancer

Dear Dr. Boston, *(I like him already. A lot of these emails start out with "Dear Sarah," which I always find strangely off-putting from someone who has never met me, because I doubt that they would address a real doctor this way.)*

My name is Marty and I am writing to you to see if you would be able to help me with my dog, Carney. She is an eight-year-old St. Bernard and she means the world to me. She was just diagnosed with bone cancer in her front leg. My vet has said that there are not a lot of good options for her and that I should put her down soon. I understand that you are doing research in osteosarcoma and I was wondering if she might be a candidate for one of your studies. I live in New York, but I am willing to travel up there to see you whenever it is convenient. I am attaching a copy of her X-rays for you to review.

Sincerely,
Marty

Subject: re: my dog with bone cancer

Dear Marty,

Thank you for your email. We would be happy to see you and Carney at our hospital and we have consultations available next Monday and Wednesday. From the X-ray that you sent, she has a very large and lytic bone lesion in her leg, which means that some of the options for limb spare are not going to be available for her. We can assess her as a candidate for limb amputation and for a clinical trial my colleague and I are doing on a new procedure called chemoembolization. With this procedure, we place a long catheter from the femoral artery to the small artery that is supplying the tumour. We give a large dose of chemotherapy through the artery that is sup- plying the tumour and then follow this with small beads that embolize, or clog up, the vessel, decreasing the blood supply to the tumour. Ideally this will give us bet- ter control of the tumour and possibly cause the tumour to shrink, or consolidate, which might make her a candi- date for limb salvage surgery.

One of our nurses will contact you to set up an appoint- ment time if you would like to come and see us.

Sincerely,

Sarah Boston, DVM, DVSc, Dipl. ACVS

I met Marty and Carney four days later. Marty drove eight hours from New York for his consultation. He was full of nervous excitement to be at our hospital. He is a big man—I mean BIG—which suited his equally big dog. Carney was a lovely St. Bernard with a big problem. Aside from her cancer, she had a lot of other orthopedic issues and was a bit overweight. We thought she might not do well on three legs (which put her in the minority of dogs). The lesion in her radius bone (just above her wrist) was so lytic (meaning the bone had been eaten away by the tumour) that it looked like it was at risk of fracturing, so radiation was not going to be a good option. The lesion was so big that a surgical limb salvage, which involves removing the tumour bone and replacing it with a metal rod (prosthesis) and a large bone plate, was not a good option either. So the owner went for the clinical trial. It would be the first time we did this procedure in a dog with osteosarcoma. In fact, as far as I knew, this was the first time that anyone in the world had done this in a dog with osteosarcoma.

Marty was all in. He was thankful and bitter at the same time: thankful that there were options for Carney and that he had found our hospital; bitter that his previous veterinarian had suggested that there were no options. Bitter, possibly approaching violent. He wanted to do everything possible for her. He let it be known that he was not happy with his previous vet and told me about his gun. I decided not to touch that one. I'm Canadian. Perhaps it was just a cultural thing. Maybe an American talking about being mad and having a gun is like a Canadian talking about making an angry phone call or writing a very stern email of complaint. He also told me that before I emailed him back, he was so miserable that he took Carney to their favourite park and held her bottle of pain medication in his hands, wondering if there was enough in there to finish him off. She was a big dog, and there were several weeks of narcotic pain medication in there, so I'm thinking, yes, that probably would have done the trick. I knew I needed to keep an eye on Marty. He spent so much time discussing death, when really the only one who was going to die was Carney. Canine osteosarcoma is a terminal disease. Marty was always lovely, grateful, and compliant with me and the staff. I really liked him and I wanted to do everything I could for him and his dog.

First, we did staging tests (chest X-rays and a bone scan) to determine if Carney had any evidence of cancer spreading to her lungs or to another bone. A bone scan involves giving the dog a radioactive drug or radioisotope intravenously. This radioisotope concentrates in areas of the skeleton where there is bone cancer. A special type of camera (called a gamma camera) is used to see where the radioisotope has accumulated, so that you can see if the bone cancer has spread to another site. Carney was negative for metastasis to her bone and to her lungs, but she had to stay in the hospital overnight after her bone scan because she was radioactive and needed to be isolated until she excreted enough of the radioactive drug to be considered safe. The regulations are different for dogs and people. A person would go home right after a bone scan, but people can self-isolate and flush their radioactive waste down the toilet. Unfortunately, animals don't have the same skill set and the radiation safety officers always have to assume the worst-case scenario: the radioactive dogs will go home, climb into bed with their owners, and urinate radioactive pee all over them and the bed.

The next morning, we used a Geiger counter to check Carney's radiation levels; her levels were low enough that she could be discharged. Marty and Carney went home for the weekend and were scheduled to come back the following week for her procedure.

I guess I forgot about the border. Maybe *forgot* is not totally accurate, because I knew that they were going back to New York, but I didn't know about the radiation portal monitors at Customs and Border Protection. At least I didn't know that they were so sensitive. It made sense after the fact, when Marty called to tell me that Carney had set off the border alarms. His vehicle had been instantly surrounded by Customs and Border Protection officers, who had their guns drawn and were demanding that he get out of the car with his hands up. More guns. Luckily, Carney was able to defuse the situation and convince the border officials that she was not a threat to national security. I was worried that Marty would be mad at me and think that I had set him up to be treated like a potential terrorist threat, but he had a good sense of humour and I think he kind of liked the border drama and the way that Carney made every single border patrol officer melt with her sweet, droopy, slobbery face.

The next week, Carney came back for her procedure. It took a long time and she was under anesthetic for most of the day. Marty sat in our waiting room for hours. He was nervous, but he had faith in our team. I had hoped to send Carney home with Marty that evening, but she was too wiped out. When I told him that she had to stay overnight, Marty was respectful, accepted this information, and took this—and every other small and big obstacle that came up—in stride.

Carney was an obliging and gentle patient. Her tail wagged constantly whenever nurses and clinicians approached her. She went home the next morning and returned two weeks later for reassessment. There was some good news; her tumour was getting smaller. This is what has been reported in people with osteosarcoma who have undergone the same procedure; it has been used to get human patients ready for limb salvage. For Carney, I was making it up as we went along. We took her to surgery and placed a bone plate that spanned above and below the tumour to try to prevent the weakened bone from breaking. Because the tumour had decreased in size, she was now a potential candidate for limb salvage with stereotactic radiosurgery, which involves giving a very high dose of radiation to the tumour, sparing the normal tissues. It is only available at certain centres with certain fancy equipment and would involve another big road trip, this time to Colorado, but there were no geographical or financial barriers for Marty. He did whatever he needed to do.

Marty brought Carney back to us after the radiation for a course of chemotherapy. Believe it or not, most dogs do very well with systemic chemotherapy. A lot of people get their ideas and images of chemotherapy from eighties and nineties movies about cancer, like *Terms of Endearment,* or one of several cancer-based movies where previously dysfunctional families must rally around Meryl Streep, or Meryl Streep must rally around her previously dysfunctional family because someone is dying of cancer. No one wants their dog to end up like Meryl Streep or Susan Sarandon circa 1998. I get that—it would be inhumane. But this passé Hollywood depiction of chemo is not what we see in most of our patients.

Carney, however, opted for the eighties Hollywood version of her treatment course. She was nauseous and ate poorly. She lost a lot of weight, which was not all bad, because she needed to lose a few pounds to take pressure off of her failing joints and her bad leg. More concerning, Carney also developed a severe infection in her leg, which was impossible to control. She had too many factors working against her. The radiation, the dead tumour bone, the bone plate, the bacteria, the chemo, and the lack of blood supply all conspired against her leg. The previous incision site from her surgery opened up, exposing the bone plate and bone. There was no option but to amputate the limb or euthanize her. Her limb salvage had failed.

Carney was given to Marty as a birthday gift when she was a puppy and, on his birthday eight years later, we amputed the leg that we had spent months, and Marty had spent thousands of dollars and miles, trying to save. It was a Saturday and we were closed except for emergencies. Marty sat in the waiting room by himself during Carney's surgery, crying. He brought up his gun again, but this time he was considering using it on himself.

Despite how awful it was for Marty to accept that Carney had to have an amputation, Carney was on a new program after her surgery. She was no longer overweight after her chemo diet, and was now free of the limb that had been bringing her down for months. Carney had finished her chemotherapy, and even though we thought she wouldn't do well on three legs, she proved us all wrong. She coped well; it just took her awhile to adjust. Marty was patient and, luckily, big enough to support her with a harness when he took her out. Within a few weeks, she was walking well on her own. Carney taught me that almost every dog can manage on three legs. We just ask an awful lot of them. We expect them to be up and walking within twenty-four hours of amputation surgery because that's the norm. But there's hope even for those dogs that aren't or can't. Most of them can still make it; it just takes more work and more patience. We would never ask so much from a person who'd undergone such a major surgery.

Carney lived for another year with minimal medical

intervention, and she enjoyed an excellent quality of life. Several times, Marty loaded her up and drove to Canada to visit us at the hospital and Carney's friends at Border Patrol.

Marty lost Carney to her disease a year and a half after her diagnosis. She lived longer than most dogs with bone cancer do, but we knew this day was coming. I worried about Marty and how he would cope. I worried that his threats of taking his own life when Carney was first diagnosed were going to come true. He did bring it up again, but he managed to come to terms with his loss. He told me that Carney's death had left a huge hole in his life, but that he would do it all again in a heartbeat because his life was so much richer for having known Carney. Ironically and sadly, Marty is now going through his own fight with cancer. True to form, he is at Sloan-Kettering, one of America's best cancer hospitals, because only the best will do for Carney and for Marty. He is fighting hard and, despite his threats to check out early, he has an intense will to live and all the strength and heart of his darling St. Bernard.

It's hard to be patient through the steps of diagnosis and treatment. It's a fine line between advocacy and being a pain in the ass, and where that line sits might just be a matter of perception. The first hurdle is finding a surgeon you can trust with yourself or your best friend. My time frame has been a bit slower than Carney's (and Marty's, I suspect, given that he is in the States), but I am going to meet my surgeon soon.

I WANTED TO SEE the best surgeon available for my thyroid mass. After almost six weeks of not-so-patiently waiting, I am finally going to meet with the head and neck surgeon in Toronto. I have played out the medical fantasy in my head many times. He will have one feel of the mass in my neck, tell me it needs to be removed immediately, admit me to the hospital, and remove the mass the next day. My medical fantasy is a reality for most of my patients. I know that it is not going to happen, but there is a small part of me that won't completely let go of the idea.

I leave the house ninety minutes before I need to, so that I am not late for my appointment. The time, date, and location of the appointment were left on my answering machine by the receptionist. It is not optional. You come at this time and date or you go to the bottom of the list. If you are late, you probably won't be seen that day, and you will go to the bottom of the list. No one will feel sorry for you, even if you might have thyroid cancer, which nobody seems to be worried about except me.

Toronto traffic and parking are a fiasco. I eventually park underground at the hospital. It is pricey but I don't care. At least I found the place and am on time. My hopeless sense of direction, my neurosis about being punctual, the dire consequences if I am not on time, and the fact that I might have cancer have all colluded to result in maximum stress levels. I am sweating.

I head up to the seventh floor for the appointment. En route, I hit every hand-sanitizing station that I pass. Human hospitals are rife with germs. I check in and sit down for a long wait. I am forty-five minutes early. The receptionist tells me that the surgeon is running a bit late because he is "in surgery." I am not sure if this is true or not because I have used that one when I am running behind. It is an indisputable, rock-solid excuse for being late when you are a surgeon. I can't do anything about the delay, so I pull out one of the many activities I have brought along for this purpose and wait. I think about what would happen if I made some of my clients wait this long; undoubtedly some of them would be marching up and down in the waiting room, demanding a face-to-face meeting with the chief of surgery, the hospital director, or the president or dean of the university—whomever they deemed to be the most powerful person in the vicinity. But today, in the human hospital, all is quiet in this very full waiting room. I guess that's why they call us patients.

Ninety minutes after my scheduled appointment time, I am moved into the examination room and told that the doctor will be with me shortly. This is good. I wait in the room for another ten or fifteen minutes. There is not much to do except stare at the diagram on the wall, which shows the anatomy of the neck and the thyroid glands in the normal and diseased states. Once the surgeon arrives, he is very nice, talks quickly, and moves fast. I like this, since I talk and move fast, too. He tells me we can

1. Try to get a new sample with a repeat ultrasound-guided aspiration of my neck. This doesn't really make sense to me as an option. It came back as benign (*didn't it?*), but it is not a very reliable test. (*And a painful neck aspiration is not ever happening again.*)

2. Leave the mass for a while and monitor it. (*I have been doing that involuntarily, and…it's growing!*)

3. Remove it and find out what it is. (*Yes! #3. I pick that one.*)

He informs me that my mass is likely benign, but believes we should take it out anyway: larger masses have more potential to be carcinoma and this one is almost 4 centimetres. I agree. I want to get it out and ask how quickly we can do it. My imaginary plan of being admitted to the hospital for surgery the next day quickly evaporates. He tells me that we will try to schedule my surgery for roughly a month from now (a month?); someone from the hospital will call me in seven to ten days to confirm the date. He hands me some forms I need to fill out: the first is a consent form. He says he will be doing the surgery, but the form says residents may also be doing things—I sign it anyway. There is also a tumour-banking form, which I sign. (We have a tumour bank where I work, too. These are repositories of tumour tissue that can be used for future cancer research, answering questions that haven't even been thought of yet. Tumour banks have been responsible for some of the most recent advances in cancer research.) One of the forms lists the potential complications that can occur during surgery: hemorrhage (bleeding); damage to the recurrent laryngeal nerve (damage to the nerve that moves your larynx, important for breathing and speaking); potential to have to convert intra-operatively from a right thyroidectomy to a complete thyroidectomy (to remove both sides of the thyroid gland and not just one, as planned), and that would, of course, double the risk of damaging one of the recurrent laryngeal nerves (then definitely won't be able to breath or talk). If both nerves are damaged, you have a tracheostomy (a big breathing hole in the neck) for the rest of your life, but the risk of that is less than 0.5 percent. My surgeon tells me that has never happened to any of his patients, and we are likely just doing one side anyway.

He then tells me that I have to go to my family doctor for a physical examination before the surgery and have him fill out another form. Nothing beyond my head and neck were examined today. I am wondering why he can't just do an examination, seeing as I am sitting right here, but this thought is interrupted by an ambush endoscope being rammed up my nose. Suddenly I am saying "eeeee" on command. He yanks the scope out of my nose, which causes a sharp pang of excruciating pain, and tells me my laryngeal function is fine.

He then starts talking even faster. There is another form for me to fill out for my pre-admission appointment, and instructions that someone will call me soon to schedule my pre-admission appointment. The plan is for me to be in the hospital overnight and to be off work for four weeks. If my mass comes back as a carcinoma, I will need the other side out in two to three months, but he suspects it will be benign. The appointment is moving fast and it seems to be wrapping up. I can't tell if he is using medical terminology for me or if he would do that anyway. It is fine for me, but I think that someone without a medical degree might be struggling to understand the surgery and risks.

He hands me his card and writes his email address on the back. Wow! I feel like a VIP, because I am pretty sure he doesn't dole out his email address to everyone, but I know his brother. I don't always give out my email to clients, but they find it anyway. They have no issue with emailing me any time, day or night. Often the emails are accompanied by an angry red exclamation point to make sure that I don't miss them and to let me know that there is nothing else more pressing in my inbox right now. The content of these emails can include lists of questions that I have already answered or will answer soon without prompting; urgent questions requiring immediate action and often emergency readmission and hospitalization of their pets (problems that require the immediacy of a phone call, not the transfer of your crisis to my inbox, which may or may not be checked until the next day); requests for consultations for pets belonging to their friends or family; and the occasional thank-you with a fantastic picture of their pet enjoying life after cancer surgery. (The last one keeps me checking my inbox.)

I thank him and feebly give him a Starbucks gift card that I made a special stop for in Guelph on the way here; that was before I arrived at the hospital to discover there was a Starbucks right in the building. So now it looks like a last-minute, amateur effort. He graciously tells me that I shouldn't have, but I explain that I wanted to thank him for his help. The whole appointment has taken twelve minutes.

I ask the receptionist for a copy of my cytology report so that I can read it on my way out. Turns out the mass is not actually benign, as I was told by my endocrinologist. The report says: "Right-sided mass: non-diagnostic sample. Left-sided mass: benign thyroid adenoma." The left side is the 1-centimetre mass that looked benign on both ultrasounds (mine and the radiologist's). The right side is the 3.8-centimetre, fast-growing mass. *Non-diagnostic* means that there were not enough cells on the slide to make a diagnosis. I know that this can happen sometimes. It's nobody's fault, but my face gets hot and my eyes fill with tears. I realize that I went through the delay and the ordeal of the painful neck aspiration for nothing and had faux-celebrated the news of the (not so) benign cytology report with my friends and family. I had used this information both to calm myself down and as validation that I had been so ridiculous all this time, thinking that I had thyroid cancer. In retrospect, the suggestion from the surgeon that we repeat the aspiration makes more sense, but I don't ever want another aspiration. I just want to move forward.

I understood almost everything that the surgeon said during my appointment, but that's because I am a surgeon. My lovely surgeon notwithstanding, the speed at which human surgeons throw information at their patients, especially people without medical training, is overwhelming. They seem to feel the need to rattle off every single possible complication and risk, just so it has all been said, no matter how remote the chance of developing this or that complication is or how much it will terrify the patient. Their patients have about as much comprehension of what has been explained to them as mine do, with the exception that my patients likely understand on some level that I love them and am trying to help them. (It is amazing how far a kiss on the head and a belly rub can go sometimes.) It's also remarkable that human patients can listen to all the potential complications but ultimately don't really have a choice in the matter: "Well, doctor, I have listened to the potential risks, and I am thinking that repairing this aortic aneurysm that is on the verge of blowing is really not for me. I am going to pass and just roll the dice out here on my own."

Two days after the consultation with my surgeon, I am doing yoga when I see another lump pop up in my neck in the mirror—this time on the other side. I investigate. It is an enlarged lymph node. Quick Google search of human lymph node anatomy and I learn that the enlarged lymph node is part of the inferior deep cervical lymph node bed. Good to know. Next, I do a quick PubMed search on thyroid carcinoma and lymph node metastasis. Normally, you would expect a right-sided tumour to spread to the lymph node on the same side, and this enlarged lymph node is on the left side. I learn that there is an 8.9 percent incidence of contralateral node metastasis with thyroid carcinoma, meaning that there is about a 9 percent chance that if your thyroid carcinoma spreads to a lymph node, it will go to the lymph node on the other side of your neck. I am freaking out again.

So, six weeks of this thyroid mass business, and now four different doctors have felt my neck and told me that the nodes are small and that is good. But now they are big and that is...bad? Just guessing. But there are other reasons for enlarged nodes. It's possible the trauma of the repeated stabbing during the time-wasting, excruciating, non-diagnostic needle biopsy could have caused reactive lymph nodes, which is just inflammation, not cancer (but that was a few weeks ago). Or I could be getting a cold (but I am not sick), or maybe it is the bubonic plague. I hear that the Bubes has made a serious comeback since we started pumping cows, dogs, and people with antibiotics, which leads to superbugs, which leads to the Bubes. (But I haven't been in a prison in Madagascar lately, so this seems less likely.) I swear I can feel the capsule that surrounds the lymph node stretching to accommodate the inflammatory cells/Bubes/cancer.

(Three days later, I feel more lymph nodes pop up on the left side, halfway up my neck. I investigate the anatomy of the human neck again. They are the superficial cervical lymph nodes. Then, another five days later, I can feel something on the other side. I can feel them all. I can feel their capsules stretching and it hurts, but it hurts on a microscopic level: microscopic aching. But I'm getting ahead of myself.)

What if it is metastasis? I had detected a mass in my thyroid early, raced home from another province to get medical attention, was patronized by a few doctors, and then slid into the lineup of the plodding Canadian health care system. What if the waiting has given it enough time to spread to my lymph nodes? Whom exactly am I supposed to sue/kill over this situation? And what am I supposed to do now? I am definitely freaking out.

I hesitate but then decide that enlarged lymph nodes are worthy of playing the VIP email card that I was given.

Subject: question — lymph nodes

Dear Dr. X,

Thank you very much for seeing me on Tuesday. It was great to meet with you and I feel very comfortable and lucky to have you as my surgeon. *(Seems a bit like I am grovelling here, totally not like me.)*

I am sorry to bother you *(with my metastatic cancer)*, but I have a question based on a change that I noticed in my neck today. This evening I noticed a small mass in the area of my left clavicle while I was doing yoga. The mass is about 0.5 cm, firm and mobile. I am concerned that it may be an enlarged lymph node. I am not as familiar with human anatomy, but it is in the area of the inferior deep cervical glands from what I can tell. This is actually on the opposite side of my thyroid mass, but I am concerned because this is a change that has occurred since I saw you.

Can you please let me know if there is anything that I should be doing about this or if it changes any of my workup?

Thank you for your help.

Sincerely,
Sarah Boston

Cell: 519-555-5239 *(In case you don't have it in the six places I wrote it and didn't catch it when I told you three times that my cell is the best way to reach me, or don't realize that a cellphone is probably the best way to reach anyone, because I would really hate to miss your call.)*

The next day:

Subject: re: question—lymph nodes

Don't think it is anything but will get an ultrasound at my hospital to assess. Emily will call you Monday with a date and time.

A

I'm very happy to have this email back, even if it is short. He is communicating with me with the brevity of a text message and I am hanging on his every character. Also, he signed it "A," which is probably because he doesn't want to waste the additional three characters on the *dam* in Adam, but also suggests that we are on a first-character basis. I wasn't sure if I could use his first name. I mean, he has a medical degree, I have a medical degree; he did a surgery residency, I did a surgery residency; he did a surgical oncology fellowship, I did a surgical oncology fellowship; he treats people with cancer, I treat dogs and cats with cancer. There it is, the glaring difference that acts as a barrier to my calling him anything but Doctor, but this email does seem like tacit approval to at least try out his first name.

Ten seconds later:

Subject: re:re: question—lymph nodes

(Was going to say Adam, but panic and just leave out any salutation or method of addressing him to be on the safe side.)

Thank you, that is great.

I will be on my cell Monday (the number that Emily reached me at before: 519-555-5239).

If I don't answer, I am in surgery but she can leave a message about when and where and I will be there. *(Because it is not as if I have a choice.)*

Thanks again,
Sarah

I get a call from his assistant, as promised, and she gives me a date for an ultrasound that is more than a month

away. This is problematic because my surgery is supposed
to be a month away, too. I try to explain the reasoning
behind the ultrasound to her: I am worried about the sud-
den appearance of enlarged lymph nodes and am feeling
a bit more urgent on this front due to said lymph nodes.
Also, the ultrasound probably needs to happen before the
surgery. She calls back again with an ultrasound appointment in ten days' time. That is the best that she can do.
Thank you, I'll be there.

Four days later:

Subject: re:re:re: question — lymph nodes

Did u get a date for an ultrasound?

Adam

One minute later:

Subject: re:re:re:re: question — lymph nodes

Hello,

Thanks so much for your email. I am booked at your hospital for an ultrasound in one week. I was going to touch
base with you to see if you thought that it was okay to
wait this long, but to be honest, I did not want to bother
you. *(As I have been reduced to a grovelling, desperate
mess by this whole process.)*

I am sure your brother told you that I am feeling pretty anxious about the whole thing and finding an enlarged lymph node has increased my stress level. *(Because I am pretty sure that this is a particularly aggressive form of metastatic thyroid carcinoma and that I am dying and no one cares.)*

I was also wondering if you are closer to knowing a surgery date (*because you said that I would have it seven to ten days from the consultation and that was over two weeks ago*), but maybe I should contact Emily about it. *(This email is obviously too long and possibly bothering you, which is a really bad idea. Sucking up to your assistant, on the other hand, seems like a really good idea, since it is likely that she is the one who holds the cards here. I probably should have given her the Starbucks gift card instead of you.)*

Thanks again for your help,
Sarah Boston

Two days later:

Subject: re:re:re:re:re: question—lymph nodes

Hi Sarah,

Ten days is fine to wait. We will figure out an exact date after your ultrasound.

Adam

Awesome. I thought this new finding would rocket me to the top of the urgent, life-saving cancer surgery list, but it has now actually set me back. I need to wait for the ultrasound date, then the results, then I can book a surgery date. Total backfire.

I go to Toronto for my ultrasound. I try to watch the ultrasound screen, but it's hard to see because I have to stretch my neck out. I also try to pump the ultrasound technician for information, but all I can get out of her is that the largest node is 1.2 centimetres in diameter, and I am not sure what this means.

Cheeky email on a Friday afternoon, two days after ultrasound:

Subject: touching base

Hi Adam *(I am now throwing out his first name like we are old friends)*,

I hope I'm not bothering you. I just wanted to check and see if you have had the opportunity to review my ultrasound report?

Thank you,
Sarah

Two days later:

Subject: re: touching base

Ultrasound looked fine. No concerning lymph nodes seen. We will just stick to our original plan.

Adam

One hour later:

Subject: re:re: touching base

Hi Adam,

Thank you so much for your email on a Sunday night. I didn't expect that, but I do appreciate it. That is great news about the ultrasound. *(Even though it was not exactly an extensive report and not sure what you mean by concerning nodes, seeing as I find it concerning that they are now palpable when they were not palpable before. One of them is 1.2 centimetres. Did you happen to notice that in your report?)*

I feel very fortunate to have you as my surgeon. *(What is wrong with me? I can't stop. I'm ridiculous.)*

I realize that the lymph node issue may have slowed things down, but do you know when I might know a surgery date? I can also contact Emily to ask her, if you would prefer.

Thanks again for your help,
Sarah Boston

Monday morning:

Subject: re:re:re: touching base

Emily should call you tomorrow or so with the date and time.

Adam

That instant:

Subject: re:re:re:re: touching base

Thank you so much.

That is great.

Cheers,
Sarah

As promised, I do get a call the next day. My surgery date is in six days' time and I have a pre-admission appointment for the next day. I have been lulled into a sluggish state because everything has been so slow, and now I need to leap into action and get myself organized for surgery in less than a week. I am happy. It is not as fast as I would have liked or as fast as I can do for my patients, but by all standards that I can measure in our health care system, it is fast and I am lucky. The pre-admission office at Women's College Hospital called me to confirm the appointment for 11 a.m. the next day. The woman I spoke to also told me several times not to be late because they go for lunch at noon. Okay, noted. I am one hour early again. I meet my pre-admission nurse. Her name is Alice, but I christen her Malice because she is really mean.

She goes through what is going to happen on the day that I am admitted. She takes my vital signs, blood pressure, height, weight, and blood. Malice shows me the requisition form with the blood tests that were ordered by my surgeon and asks me if I can read the last word. I can't decipher it either and she shrugs and moves on. I hope it wasn't important, because I guess I am not having that test done. I think about some of the recent reading I have done on medical error and communication failures in human surgery. I tell her about my medical history and have brought her information from my family doctor, including two very minor medical conditions that I know will not cause any issues with my anesthesia or surgery, but one of them is related to my heart. I have a small atrial septal defect and recently had a stress test, a cardiac ultrasound, and wore a Holter monitor. It has never caused a problem and likely never will. She thinks it would be a good idea for me to see an anesthesiologist today, just in case.

She then asks if I have questions and I ask her if it is women only at Women's College Hospital. In an effort to entertain myself and to ward off the stress and Malice's malevolence, I start to daydream that Women's College Hospital was built by women for women. It still looks like a hospital, but with better lighting and decor and more mirrors. It smells like Bath & Body Works and is staffed with cool nurses who have body piercings, swirly floral tattoos and trendy hair, and are wearing a combination of scrubs and lululemon. The whole place has the feeling of a cross between a womyn's folk festival and an episode of *Nurse Jackie*. Spontaneous yoga and deep girl-on-girl hugging is breaking out in the halls. The patients are women with female-specific cancers and other female-only ailments and they are recovering from their treatments together in sisterly solidarity.

Malice snaps me back to the present and pops my girl-power bubble by telling me that the hospital recently reorganized and now focuses on day procedures; the majority of treatments are for orthopedics (on mostly men) and for male infertility (ironic). Apparently they don't have in-patients any more (except me). I am shattered. At the very least I was hoping that my insurance-covered semi-private room would come equipped with a roomie who had a shared experience. Maybe she would even have had a thyroidectomy on the same day and we could bond over our missing thyroids, the thin and ineffective hospital blankets, pee breaks, sleep interruptions, and potent narcotics, while strategizing ways to cover our neck scars.

I then ask Malice if she saw the form that says I can have a semi-private room with my insurance and she snorts and says, "Yeah, we will put you where we put you because we don't have in-patients here any more."

"Except for me," I mutter.

"And you will be lucky to have a bed. You will probably be recovering in the emergency room."

There she is mistaken, because if I find myself recovering in a big-city emergency room full of the noise and din of the endless drama of late-night human misery, pestilence, injury, and disease, I will be getting into a cab and recovering in a nearby hotel. I ask her when visiting hours are and she tells me she has no idea because they reorganized the hospital in September (eight months ago) and they don't have in-patients any more (except for me) so she can't really answer this outlandish question, which has clearly come out of left field. I am thinking that Malice did not fare too well with the not-so-recent hospital reorganization; her disdain for her new role as pre-admissions nurse is as palpable as my neck lump and lymph nodes. Thanks, Malice, you have painted a lovely picture of my recovery as I struggle to find myself a bed in a busy ER, surrounded by big-city traumas and lame, impotent, infertile men, with no prospect of quiet, warmth, dark, semi-privacy, or even a visit from my husband.

She then leaves to find out when the anesthesiologist can see me. It is around 11:15 a.m. She says he is busy until after 1 p.m. and tells me to come back at 1 p.m. I ask her if I need to be back at exactly 1 p.m. because I was hoping to go meet my friend for lunch. She tenses and quips that it is really not appropriate for me to be going for lunch with my girlfriend when she is trying to help me and set up a time for an anesthesiologist to see me (two hours from now) and it is for my own safety that I need to be back at 1 p.m. sharp. I guess it is pretty selfish of me to want to see my friend before I have cancer surgery. What was I thinking? I don't have time to see my friend and get back in time, so I go and eat crappy fast food by myself in the food court of the nearest mall. I get back at exactly 1 p.m. as ordered and sit in the waiting room until the anesthesiologist can see me — at 2:15 p.m.

He is pleasant but seems a bit bewildered (as am I) as to why he is seeing a thirty-seven-year-old, completely healthy (minus the cancer) woman with normal blood work and a minor congenital heart defect that has never caused a clinical problem and was fully worked up by a cardiologist within the past year. He does, however, seem genuinely chuffed that I am a veterinary surgeon and he asks me how hard it is to place an endotracheal tube in a cat. I think he likes cats. I tell him that cats are pretty easy, but rabbits are nearly impossible to intubate and that he is welcome to visit our veterinary teaching hospital some time if he wants to see the procedure for himself. He is completely captivated by the rabbit fact.

He starts to take a look at me, and grabs a stethoscope that is broken on one side. The tube is disconnected from the earpiece. I am not sure if I should say anything, but I am certain that he will not hear a thing. He mutters that he doesn't really know why he is listening to me anyway when he has a full report from a cardiologist on his desk, but he goes through the motions. The optics are better, considering that I have been waiting for him for nearly three hours now. He puts the scope on my chest, waits, and hears nothing. I try not to laugh. He looks down and realizes the scope has had it. He aborts the mission and again states that he doesn't really need to listen to me anyway. I tell him that I puke on Demerol, which he agrees is nasty stuff. I also tell him that I am always cold. I am more concerned about nausea and hypothermia than I am about pain or death. I ask him if he will be the anesthesiologist on Monday and he says he is off clinics on Monday, so someone else will take care of me, making this consultation with him even less valuable. There is not really much more to say, so I thank him for his time and head out. Bye -bye, Malice, see you next week.

I WASN'T SURE WHAT to expect from the appointment with my surgeon. All I really had to go on was my own experience of seeing patients. Some things were similar and some were very different. The wait-time-to-appointment-length ratio was different. I would say that my experience in the human world was 5:1, five time units of waiting to one time unit spent with my doctor. In the veterinary world, it is more like 1:5. Even a wait of fifteen to twenty minutes will cause clients to visibly tense up and look at their watch when I enter the exam room. I always smile big, apologize for the wait, and get started. I know I will win them over, it is just a matter of time.

The parking situation at a veterinary university teaching hospital is similarly shameful to the parking situation at a human hospital. Just to fuel the client's anxiety even further, we have parking meters that must be fed every hour, so while clients wait for us, they can mark the passing time with the aggravation that they need to keep getting more change to feed the meters or they will get a ticket.

The one striking similarity between appointments with human or veterinary surgeons is the anxiety. I understand the anxiety now in a way that I never did before. I have been the client before and taken my own pets to see the vet, which is a good lesson in empathy, but now I have also been the patient. Anxiety can do strange things to the behaviour of perfectly normal people. Most of the anxiety comes from having absolutely no idea what to expect. Many pet owners try to control their anxiety with lists of questions, calling and emailing ahead of time and trying to get a pre-consultation consultation. In an effort to educate the masses and demystify the appointment with a veterinary surgical oncologist, this is a list of frequently asked questions taken from my real life.

Frequently Asked Questions

Pre-operative questions

When will my dog have surgery?

We usually do pre-operative tests like ultrasounds, X-rays, and CT scans on the same day as the appointment and then admit our patients for surgery the day after. Some people are disappointed that surgery does not happen on the same day. They are further disappointed that their dog is not ready to go home the evening after a full diagnostic workup and major surgery. Others are shocked that things happen so fast. These people have usually spent time in the human system and all they are expecting from their surgery consultation is a consultation. What my clients don't know is that the plan to admit my patients for surgery the next day is my own failed fantasy for myself.

Will my dog have to stay overnight? Can I sleep in his kennel with him?

The truth is, there are a couple of veterinary referral hospitals in the world that can accommodate this request, but I don't work at one of them. Some of my clients are so distraught at the thought of leaving their dog overnight before surgery that they are willing to drive several hours to take their dog home that evening, often after a general anesthetic or sedation, and then get up at 5 a.m. or earlier to be back in time for surgery early the next morning. We are supposed to admit our patients overnight to ensure that they have fasted and are ready to undergo general anesthesia in the morning. My efforts to stick to this rule and admit my patients the night before surgery have become weaker and more pathetic over time. I usually relent and just admit them the morning of surgery, because that is easier than trying to explain why a person cannot sleep in a dog run at a veterinary hospital and because I wouldn't want to leave my dog overnight either if I didn't have to. I would be too sad.

How many stitches will my dog have?

People get hyper-focused on the number of stitches it takes to close an incision, like it is a badge of honour to have lots of stitches. I have never counted the number of sutures that I put in, so I don't know how many I will give your dog. I can probably tell you how long the incision will be. And while we are on that topic, I should also tell you that most tumour removals are circular incisions that are closed in a straight line, which leads to something we call dog ears (pun intended), where the ends of the incision have little peaks or ears. You can correct them by removing more tissue, but I usually don't do that because (1) it will make the incision longer, which will mean more stitches, (2) I am lazy, and (3) they will flatten out over time and the incision will heal and hair will grow over it. (*Warning: lame vet joke ahead.*) Your dog is not going to be a bikini model any more. I had one client, who was a dental nurse, scream at me on the phone for over an hour because of the way her obese corgi looked with his dog ears. Her dog had two malignant tumours removed (and cured, I would like to add), but because he was so fat, the incisions were deep and the dog ears were very dramatic. But even his crazy-ass devil horns flattened over time, so if they can, your dog's will be fine, too.

Will my dog be disfigured?

Your dog has a big tumour, which is disfiguring in its own right. The surgery to remove it may also alter his appearance, but dogs have hair and they don't care. Everyone wants the tumour to be gone so that their dog will look completely normal and everything can go back to normal. This may or may not be possible; it depends what the tumour is and where it is located.

Can you trim his nails and express his anal sacs while he is here?

Yes, as a board-certified veterinary surgeon with fellowship training in surgical oncology, I would be more than happy to perform the same duties as your dog groomer. Expressing anal sacs is a particularly enjoyable task, and I would love to do it at no extra charge.

Can you clean his teeth while he is under anesthetic?

Your dog is here for major cancer surgery. It is not a good idea to combine surgery with his prophylactic dental cleaning and I don't do this because I am a cancer surgeon *(see above)*.

Random questions that have nothing to do with the current appointment

Do you stick your arm up cows' bums?

You would be amazed at how often I get asked this question. Usually, the person is snickering when they ask, but little do they know it takes a good six to eight years of higher education to acquire this skill. The first thing you have to learn is how to do it without laughing, which takes practice. I never wanted to learn, but I had no choice. There was no streaming into large animal and small animal medicine when I was a vet student, so you had to learn everything. To say I learned all of it might be a bit generous. I spent more time grooming my palpation cow in vet school than I did putting my arm up her bum, because, to be honest, I felt like I was anally raping her, and reproduction was not my strong suit in vet school or in life. I understood very little about why I was putting my arm up there and for what I was supposed to be feeling. For the record, my husband has since taught me that you are usually feeling for ovaries to see where the cow is in her cycle so you know when to breed her. So, yes, I have stuck my arm up a cow's bum, but no, I do not do it any more. There is just not a lot of call for that sort of thing in the small animal referral hospital where I work.

I wanted to be a veterinarian but I didn't think I could put animals down. How do you do it?

This is one of the most common questions I get asked about being a veterinarian. There is a bit of tone there, suggesting that maybe I am the one with the problem. I have the recessive kill-pets gene, which allows me to kill beloved family pets effortlessly. I am not sure why there is a morbid fascination with putting animals down. No one wants to do this—it's never fun. Sometimes it's okay, sometimes it's really hard, and sometimes you just can't do it. Most veterinarians are focused on keeping animals alive and healthy. (I always thought that a veterinary practice limited to euthanasia would never fly as a business model, but there is one in Florida and it's thriving.)

Do you have to be good at science and math to be a veterinarian?

I think this is probably the biggest reason that a lot of people give up their childhood dream of becoming a veterinarian, even though most people cite that it is because they could never put animals down. Science and math are fairly important in pursuing a medical degree, even if you are just a doggie doctor.

Random questions that are loosely associated with the current appointment

Have you heard about this new cancer diet (name of some absurd canine cancer diet from the Internet) or holistic cure (pick any herbal medication at random)? It was clinically proven to cure cancer. Do you want me to print out the information for you so you can learn about it?

When I tell clients that I have not heard about the diet or holistic cure, they always seem a bit disappointed in me and worried that I might not know what I am doing. Everyone tries to find an Internet cure when they are dealing with a cancer diagnosis. But don't you think that if there were a real cure for cancer on the Internet (1) it would would not be so secret, and (2) I would know about it?

What presents should I buy for you? Can I cook for you?

Our clients are notoriously generous. Usually there is a lot of food involved. The oncology department is the food hub of any veterinary referral hospital. For the record, my favourite present is the always fashionable Starbucks gift card. You cannot beat a guilt-free five-dollar steamy milk beverage. To answer the second question, I am going to say no. Please do not cook for me. I have a lot of clients who kindly devote their time to baking or cooking for us. On more than one occasion, I have been presented with a Crock-Pot full of stew. It is a challenging gift to eat on the fly in a busy animal hospital. We just don't have the facilities to accommodate a sit-down stew meal in the middle of our day. Also, I don't eat meat. But the bigger problem is my OCD tendencies, which I come by honestly as a surgeon. Whenever food is brought in that was not made in an industrial, regularly inspected, government-regulated commercial kitchen, I cannot eat it, no matter how hungry I am. As soon as I look at that slow cooker full of stew or that plate of homemade cookies, my mind will simultaneously flash to the six dirtiest kitchens I have ever seen, a cat crapping in a litter box and then jumping up on the kitchen counter and/or sampling stew from the pot, and the bathroom line at Disney World, where I observed that the rate of handwashing was less than 50 percent. I am sorry. You are so generous, and I appreciate the effort and the thought, but I just can't eat the stew.

Are we best friends now?

Wow, this is awkward. I'm sorry, but the answer is no. We are friendly, but you are my client, so we can't be friends. We have a professional relationship right now. Are you friends with your dentist? I didn't think so. Why would you be? I know it is confusing because I am spending so much time with you and your lovely dog and we are going through this emotional time together, and no one else really understands you and how much you love your dog. Also, I know that I am quite cool and you imagine that hanging out with me would be awesome (it is), and being friends with me would also be a ticket to free veterinary advice, which would be nice for you, but we can't be friends. No exceptions. Except maybe Ellen DeGeneres; I would let her be my friend if she were a client. Ellen, if you are reading this: (1) I am grateful, and (2) yes, I will let you be my friend, thanks for asking.

Can I call you Sarah?

I don't really care, but if you are asking, I prefer Dr. Boston (*see above, professional relationship/dentist/Ellen*), but it's not that important to me. I actually prefer Sarah to Dr. Sarah because Dr. Sarah seems cute and diminutive, like you don't think I am a real doctor. I should call this an infrequently asked question, now that I think about it, because no one ever asks. They just call me Sarah.

If it looks bad in there will you just go ahead and euthanize him?

I'm not sure where this question comes from. The answer is no, that will never happen. I can't just euthanize your dog without talking to you. I will never come out after surgery, tear off my surgery cap, shake my head, hit the wall dramatically, and say "Goddammit!" under my breath, and then tell you that it was bad in there, real bad, and I made the decision to surprise-euthanize your dog. A more likely scenario would be that if things look bad, I call you and *you* may decide to put *your* dog down without recovering him from surgery.

Questions that I am not going to answer, hoping that the lack of response gives you the message. (Hint: the answer is no.)

Are you going to do experiments on my dog in the back?

Can I have your personal cellphone number so that I can contact you any time, day or night?

Is that a smartphone and will you receive and respond to all of my email messages instantly?

I know you said that I should come at 6:00 p.m. to pick up my dog so you can get home before 7:00, but I can't make it there until 9:00 tonight, 9:30 at the latest, unless I hit traffic, then it might be a bit later. Is that okay?

Post-operative questions

How long will it be until my dog will have his next solid, anally satisfying bowel movement? When would it be appropriate to bust out the suppositories if this is not happening?

I have never understood the level of focus on when a dog will poo post-operatively. If they are pooping on schedule, it means all is well in the world again. Many clients are also very quick to administer suppositories to get things going. The first time I had a client tell me that they gave their dog a suppository, I had to excuse myself from the exam room so I could go and look up the word *suppository*. Anyone who is helping out their dog in this way must have self-suppository-administering experience, and here is where I need us to stop talking about it.

When can my dog go to the groomer and/or have a bath?

A lot of our clients will get their dogs groomed before their appointments, which is so adorable and considerate! We will take that lovely grooming job and shave half of it and get blood on the other half, but that is okay, it is all going to be fine. Give it two weeks before a bath.

Questions that break my heart

Did I do something to cause my dog's cancer?

This is often the hidden cause of a lot of the anxiety — people are worried that they are crappy dog owners (or that I am going to think that they are crappy dog owners) because they did something wrong or neglectful and they caused their dog to get cancer. Everyone wants to find a reason or a cause for cancer. Everyone wants something to blame, even if it is themselves. Generally, no, we don't always know what causes cancer. Except for a small number of very specific causes, it is usually nothing that anyone did or didn't do. Unless your dog has been working with asbestos or smoking — then it is all your fault.

How much will it cost? Do you have a payment plan?

If clients cannot afford treatment, this question is always accompanied by a devastating amount of guilt and shame. It is okay, really; not everyone can afford this type of care. When clients don't have the financial wherewithal to treat, it is heartbreaking for everyone and causes major conflict for all veterinarians. There is a side of me that sees a pet as a luxury item and a hobby (I see having children in the same way), and the reality is that luxury items and hobbies are expensive, so people who choose to have them should be prepared with a big disposable income or pet insurance. (Children are hobbies with hobbies; the compounded expenses of this endeavour boggles my mind.) The other side of me just cannot take being told one more time that vets are too expensive by someone who smokes, drives an expensive car, plays golf, goes on beach holidays each year, has a huge new flat-screen TV or a new kitchen, a twice-a-day latte habit, a new iPhone 12 and iPad 9 for each family member, or a thousand-dollar purse. I find that invalidating. It is, however, truly painful to see a family with a pet that they dearly love who have the desire, but not the financial means, to treat.

Can you cure him?

Sometimes, yes. Sometimes you can cure cancer with surgery if you can cut it all out and it hasn't spread. That is what I find so intoxicating about cancer surgery: it has the potential to cure the disease.

If he needs blood, can I give him my blood? Or a more extreme variation: Can I donate one of my kidneys or part of my liver to my dog?

These clients go beyond just spending thousands of dollars and all of their time. They are willing to give blood or an organ if it will save their dog's life. It's a whole new level of commitment. So, the answer is no: it wouldn't work for you to give your kidney or a lobe of your liver to your dog because it would be rejected, because you are human and your dog is a dog, but great question.

Most of my clients are dream clients. They are sweet, appreciative, educated about veterinary health, and willing to do anything and everything for their dog. They apologize for being stressed, for their cellphone ringing, for crying, for being late, or any other inconvenience that they may have caused. They drive for hours for appointments and procedures, wait for hours during diagnostics and treatments, and never complain. They put their lives on hold for their dog's care. I've had clients who have moved to town temporarily to be closer to the hospital where their pet is being treated. They don't seem fazed by the thousands of dollars they are spending. They just shrug and say things like, "It is what it is," or "It has to be done," or "What else are you going to do?" as they sign the quote.

I had a client from Buffalo with a dog name Moses and another dog named Eli. Moses had a massive skull tumour that was too big for surgery. He needed a special type of radiation. It was late December. The owner left town on December 23 and drove Moses to Colorado for treatment so he could get the dog in during the window of time between Christmas and New Year's. Then he drove back over New Year's. He missed Christmas and New Year's with his family. He came in for a recheck when he got back and I asked him about his trip and missing Christmas. I assumed he was Jewish because he had dogs named Moses and Eli and seemed to have no qualms about skipping Christmas. Nope, he wasn't Jewish, and he was married and had a four-year-old daughter. He tried to trick his daughter into thinking Christmas was on the twenty-second of December that year, but she was nobody's fool.

My clients forever humble me. How do they do it? The supply of time, money, and love seems endless. Even moving Christmas one year is not too much to ask for a dog named Moses.

TODAY THE OPERATING ROOM tables are turned. The surgeon is having, not doing, surgery. To be clear, a dog is not doing surgery on me, so I guess the tables are not literally turned. That would be ridiculous and would require a very well-trained and focused dog. The tables are turned, nonetheless, because I am a veterinary surgical oncologist and I am having surgery today to remove a mass in my thyroid. The irony of this is not lost on anyone, so I might as well just acknowledge it. Yes. Very ironic that someone who works with cancer would get cancer, or at least have a cancer scare. And yes, also ironic that I am having a procedure that I have done many times. My patients are dogs, though, and they don't need to be able to talk or work post-operatively, so that is one subtle but important difference. My patients only know that they are away from home, spending time in a cage, and people are poking them. They don't know that they are having surgery, that bad things could happen, or that the lump in their neck that everyone keeps feeling could be very bad news. Lucky them.

Past events at the veterinary teaching hospital where I work add an extra chill to this irony. Three years ago, a close colleague and one of my mentors, a fifty-eight-year-old cardiovascular surgeon, died of a heart attack while he was sleeping. Recently, another colleague and dear friend who was a veterinary neurologist at our hospital died of a brain aneurysm. Although this is clearly not as dramatic, my colleague and friend who is an orthopedic surgeon has had no less than five knee surgeries to try to correct a cruciate injury. One of the pioneers of renal disease in dogs recently had her kidney removed. And now the cancer surgeon has a mass in her neck and needs a cancer surgeon to remove it. It's spooky. I have started to wonder if my teaching hospital is cursed; it seems to me that if you work here, you either get the disease you study and treat or you have twins. (There is a strangely high incidence of twins among my co-workers.) Hmm, thyroid mass or twins? I'm going to have to think about that one. Let me sketch it out (see table 1).

Table 1: Similarities between twin pregnancy and thyroid cancer due to veterinary teaching hospital employee curse

Pregnant with Twins	Thyroid Tumour
Initiating event (fertilization) causes rapid, exponential growth of a mass of cells	Initiating event (carcinogensis) causes rapid, exponential growth of a mass of cells
People want to touch it	People want to touch it

Pregnant with Twins	Thyroid Tumour
Requires removal and after-care	Requires removal and after-care
One of the only ways to get any time off work	One of the only ways to get any time off work
People anxious to know their names	People anxious to know diagnosis
Potential to behave badly and kill you	Potential to behave badly and kill you
Can cause drastic appearance change and weight gain	Can cause drastic appearance change and weight gain
Life-altering	Life-altering

I arrive early to check in to the hospital. Soon I am taken to the back with a nurse to change into a hospital gown and to put everything I brought with me into a big plastic bag with my name on it. She is really kind and she gives me a pre-warmed blanket and housecoat when I tell her that I am always cold. I am relieved. I head to the waiting room and wait to be called. A man and his two kids are sitting nearby. I gather from his conversation with a very earnest and eager volunteer that his wife is still in surgery, and I overhear that we have the same surgeon, which leads me to believe that until she comes back with another cheery update, I am not going anywhere. Good to know. It's a little surprising that they use volunteers to keep patients' families and patients informed on their surgery day. I can't imagine ever handing this task over to a volunteer for my own clients. I wouldn't trust them, and my clients would never tolerate it.

More waiting. I see Malice cross the waiting room, bringing more patients to her office to scare them in her confidence-stripping pre-admission horror show. I hide under my blanket. I can't deal with Malice today. I think she might eat my soul. The earnest volunteer is working the room with her clipboard and her comfortable shoes and support hose. She tells the family that the surgery on their wife/mother is almost over and everything is fine. My turn soon.

I am taken from the general waiting room to a separate holding area for patients only, which is directly outside the operating rooms. A nurse quickly goes over my history. She leaves me and I see my friend the anesthesiologist from last week. He comes over and tells me that I am in good hands today with his colleague, and then he gets my email address because he really does want to visit our veterinary teaching hospital at some point. Then another nurse goes over a checklist with me. I quietly thank Atul Gawande for writing *The Checklist Manifesto*, which emphasizes surgical pre-planning. I find it comforting that everyone knows who I am and what body part to remove.

The anesthesia resident comes to talk to me. She is fresh meat. Given the time of year, I would not be surprised if she's just graduated from medical school and this is the first week of her residency. I might even be one of her first patients. She looks more nervous than I am. I tell her that I puke and get cold easily, which is what I tell everyone who is taking care of me, because I am so worried about it and hoping someone will listen. She tells me it should all be good because we are using TIVA today. I ask her what that stands for and she panics. She has no idea. So I ask her what drugs are being used. Nothing. I tell her I am just asking because I am a veterinary surgical oncologist. This makes things worse. She starts stuttering and is back to grasping for the meaning of her acronym, "Total Intra...?"

"Total intravenous anesthesia?" I say, finishing her sentence. Not very reassuring. Baby resident goes away with her tail between her legs.

My surgeon and his fellow drop by to say hi. We go over another quick checklist and he writes on the right side of my neck with a marker, which is protocol, but it is fairly obvious which side needs to come out; the huge mass sticking out is a dead giveaway. I make another plea for a warm, puke-free recovery, and add a request for a little extra care on the closure of the surgical site to avoid having a big scar on my neck. Since vanity is the whole reason that I found this mass in the first place, there is no point in pretending. I'm vain. The neck is pretty close to the face. I would prefer the no-scar option. I know that the amount of care taken with the suturing and surgical technique will make the difference between a faint scar that only I can see and a big fat cheloid mess, just below my face. My surgeon looks a bit irritated by the question and he tells me that the incision has to be as big as the mass is to get it out. I know that, but I'm not talking about the length of the incision, I am talking about closing the incision so it doesn't scar. Then I stop talking because they are walking away and heading toward the OR.

The nurse comes back one more time to take me into the operating room. The anesthesiologist, who will be supervising the baby resident, takes the opportunity to introduce herself as I walk in. I am relieved. I think she is trying to win back my confidence after realizing her resident is unable to name basic anesthetic drugs or remember what TIVA stands for. I get on the table. Baby resident is now going to try her luck at putting an IV catheter in my hand. She might be an IV virgin; I get this impression because she is fumbling and seems to have no idea where to put it. She tries every angle to direct the catheter to the correct place, except for the direction in which the vein happens to be running. It hurts a lot. The anesthesiologist, seeing this distinct lack of technical prowess, bumps her baby resident out of the way, removes the catheter from my now very bruised hand and places another catheter at a different site, all in about ten seconds. Baby resident is now coming at me with a syringe. I am not sure what it contains and neither is she, but she is going to give it to me anyway. She tells me that it is my "welcome cocktail" and in it goes and then...

Blackness for an undetermined period of time.

"She's falling!" I'm falling. Hands are catching me and I am hoisted up and onto a bed.

More blackness.

I am now in recovery. Shannon, the recovery nurse, asks me if I want some fentanyl (an opioid that is related to morphine). Yes, is my reflexive response; it seems appropriate given the circumsances. I am in pain and not in pain at the same time. I am trying to talk to her and remember her name but I am slipping in and out of consciousness.

"Shannuhhnn, did they drop me?"

I can't figure out if that happened or not.

I refocus, deciding that I will never know. Shannon is

not talking. I suddenly remember what Malice told me about the hospital reorganization and the lack of beds and that they would put me wherever they have space. I could be recovering in the ER with infertile men. I panic. As much as someone who is on a lot of narcotics and sedatives can panic.

"Shannon, please don't send me to the emergency room to recover. Can you find me a room?" She has now decided that I am crazy and assures me I will not be recovering in the emergency room; no, they did not drop me; and they are finding me a room and a bed. This all comes as a huge relief. I fall back into my narcotic-induced sleep state.

Darkness.

Next thing I know two porters are wheeling me and my big plastic bag of belongings down the hall—to my very own room—husband in tow. They are telling me jokes the whole way. One is about the pope and the other one is about some guy who goes to the emergency room with lettuce sticking out of his ass. This leads me to panic again, thinking that I will be recovering in the emergency room beside some weirdo who sticks vegetables in his anus. I have a friend who is an ER doctor. Things like this happen all the time. One of the porters tells me the doctor said the case was just the "tip of the iceberg," and they both start laughing. I realize that there is no lettuce-ass guy in the ER.

I am wheeled into a small private room with its own bathroom. The room is very warm and my nurse is a lovely woman from Trinidad with a cool patois that makes me feel relaxed. The fact that I am stoned out of my gourd also promotes this feeling of relaxation. Life is good. I am pain-free and euphoric and very aware of the fact that the mass in my neck that has been driving me crazy is gone. Not that I can touch my neck, because everything is too swollen and it would hurt too much, but the knowledge that the mass is not there is a huge relief. My surgeon swings by to see me and tells me that things went well and that the mass looked benign, which is nice, but I don't believe him. The hydromorphone is good and I am up most of the night sending sassy text messages to friends and watching the details of yet another Canadian federal election as it plays out on my iPad. I am riveted. It is hard to sleep because I am on a drug schedule that requires a treatment every two hours, and the lights are on, and I am too immobile to turn them off, and too stoned to think to ask someone to do that for me.

At some point, I realize that my upper lip is really swollen and there is a big cut inside it. I deduce that this is most likely the result of the baby anesthesia resident trying her unskilled hand at placing the endotracheal tube. She likely caught my upper lip around my front teeth as she pulled my upper jaw back with the instrument that is used to pull the palate out of the way during intubation, driving my front teeth through my lip in the process. It will go nicely with the massive bruise on my hand. I also realize that my throat is sore and there is an abrasion on the roof of my mouth. I suspect that the intubation went about as smoothly as the IV catheter placement, but someone must have gotten it in because I am still here.

I am also on a drug called ondansetron, which is a potent anti-nausea drug used for chemotherapy patients. Either my surgeon or the anesthesiologist put me on it immediately, without waiting for me to be nauseous. All my pleas for a nausea-free recovery have paid off. I am not even a little bit nauseous. I feel great. I think back to when I had my gallbladder out eleven years ago and how I was puking and crying because of the nausea. I had told them I was nauseous before the projectile puking, but no one treated me until it was too late. They didn't listen. The difference is night and day. I start to wonder how many of my patients wake up nauseous. It is hard to gauge nausea in veterinary patients until it is really bad. There are so many reasons why a dog or a cat might curl up and sit at the back of the cage after surgery and refuse to eat or drink. Pain? Cold? Fear? Exhaustion? Trying to sleep? Depression? Loneliness? Nausea? When the nausea gets really bad, they will drool a lot and start retching, but then it is too late. They're miserable. You can see it on their faces. I am suddenly inspired to research this and design a randomized, blinded prospective clinical trial evaluating the use of anti-nausea medication to treat post-operative nausea and vomiting in veterinary patients. I grab my iPad and start writing. I don't want to forget this idea. These are some good drugs I'm on.

The next morning, the nurse and surgeon check me over and I am deemed good to go. One more dose of hydromorphone for the road and I am out the door. I am still stoned and sending triumphant texts to my friends about my excellent choice of post-operative outfit—velour Juicy Couture loungewear—as I head home.

Once home, and approximately four hours after my last dose of hydromorphone, the fun stops. My euphoria is gone and replaced by pain and sadness. I am falling a second time, but there is no one to catch me.

I recover at home in bed for two weeks. I thought I would do some cool things on my sick leave, but I can't even focus enough to watch a movie. It is great to get some paid time off, but the real downside of sick leave is that you are sick. The Tylenol 3s are okay, except they don't really take away all the pain and they give me heartburn. I want to get off them as soon as I can. I know I need to stop taking codeine if I want to think clearly, stay awake, gain control of my emotions, or ever poo again. I am knocked on my ass by this experience much more than I expected. My only reference is my thyroid cancer patients. I am not the happy dog who is dragging me down the hall by his leash and telling his owner the whole story in the barking song of the reunited the day after surgery.

I am full of respect and awe for my patients. They sail through their surgeries with dignity and grace. They make no complaints and have endless forgiveness for the things we do to them. All they ask in return is a bit of hand-feeding and some human kindness.

Woof!

IT'S HARD TO COMPARE a dog's experience of cancer surgery to that of a person. A few things make it easier on them: first, they don't know that they have cancer, and second, they have less time to think about the fact that they have cancer (if they could know that they have cancer in the first place) because they move through the process so much faster. Some things are harder. I wish I could explain to them what we are doing, why we are poking them, why they wake up in pain, and why they are sleeping in a cage. It's heartbreaking if I think about it too much. Most of my patients are used to sleeping in a bed every night with their owners. The cage and the solitude must be very confusing. Even for the same surgical procedure, the experience for the human and animal patient is worlds apart.

Once, when I was out of town at a veterinary conference, I got a customary email from my surgical oncology intern with a run down of our cases.

Subject: checking in

Hi Sarah,

I hope the conference was good. This is an update on our guys:

Logan: decubital ulcer developed on contralateral elbow after forelimb amputation. *(Translation: a full-thickness pressure sore has developed on his elbow after his other leg was amputated.)* Plan is to manage with bandage changes and recheck in seven days. Chemotherapy is postponed until the wound has healed.

Daisy: Hemipelvectomy with multiresistant post-operative wound infection. Systemically well and has responded to vacuum-assisted closure. *(Translation: a dog that has had half the pelvis and accompanying limb removed and subsequently developed a multiresist-ant bug is responding to wound therapy.)* Discharged this week. Histo shows low-grade sarcoma with clean margins.

Lily: ten-year-old female cat with a history of respiratory distress. Thoracic rads show large mediastinal mass. Cytology consistent with thymoma. CT shows mass is large but appears resectable, no mets. *(Translation: chest X-rays and CT scan show a large mass in the chest. Needle biopsy is consistent with a thymoma. It looks big but also looks like it can be removed with surgery.)* The owner is currently undergoing

chemotherapy for metastatic colon cancer. Will be in
next week for a surgery consult with you.

Jake: nine-year-old male castrated German shepherd
cross with a mandibular mass. Thoracic rads, CT of head
and thorax performed. Negative for mets. *(Translation: chest X-rays and CT scan of the head and chest
have been done. No evidence of spread.)* Owners very
stressed but want to treat. Coming in next week for
mandibulectomy *(surgery to remove the tumour and
part of the jaw)*.

Lulu: twenty-nine-year-old woman, history of possible cystitis and left cranial abdominal pain. Seen at
Guelph General. Suspected possible pyelonephritis as
no response to two courses of antibiotics and increasing levels of abdominal pain. Abdominal ultrasound
showed 9-cm cavitated splenic mass. Confirmed by CT
scan. *(Translation: suspected kidney infection has not
responded well to antibiotics, and increasing levels of
pain. Abdominal ultrasound and CT scan showed a 9
cm mass in the spleen.)* Patient is in a lot of pain and
awaiting further work up and treatment.

My intern has a pretty wild sense of humour. When she
describes Lulu, she is, of course, describing herself. Like a
lot of people in Ontario, she doesn't have a family doctor
and was trying to get a referral to a surgeon through one of
the many ER doctors she has seen over the past two weeks.

An ultrasound was done to evaluate her kidneys. The
excruciating pain that the ultrasound probe caused when

it was pushed against her abdomen, combined with the look on the ultrasound technician's face and the image that was left on the screen when the technician excused herself to get the radiologist to "check the images" were all pretty telling that something was seriously wrong, even to a layperson. But Lulu is not a layperson; she is a veterinarian. She could see on the screen that there was a large mass in her abdomen. The radiologist came back and imaged it herself, which is also a sign that things are not good. Radiologists rarely do their own ultrasounds in human medicine. She was admitted overnight and had a CT scan the next day.

She was discharged by an emergency doctor after the CT scan. As the doctor was shuffling Lulu out the door, Lulu asked, "What is the chance that this thing is going to rupture?"—which is our biggest concern with splenic masses in dogs. Not that it's the same thing; splenic masses in dogs have a much higher chance of being malignant. In humans, most splenic masses are benign. Lulu may or may not have known this. She was working on a research project on splenic lymphoma, which is eerie and made me worry that she had developed splenic lymphoma because of the curse. Veterinarians would be more prone to head straight to surgery to get the spleen out of there. It doesn't really matter if it is benign or malignant—a big, painful splenic mass that might rupture and hemorrhage needs to be treated with a splenectomy.

The rupturing comment made the ER doc pause. She postponed Lulu's discharge for a bit while she called surgeons for advice and enacted a plan. She transferred the case to a hospital in Hamilton and told Lulu that someone would call her in a few days to set up an appointment with a surgeon. Lulu asked if she should get her CT and ultrasound images uploaded to a CD and take it with her to the surgeon. The ER doctor told her that she would send it all over with her referral and not to worry. She sent Lulu home. It was Friday, July 13.

Lulu spoke with the surgeon's surly assistant on July 18 and was told that the next appointment with the surgeon was July 30. She was beside herself; her abdominal pain had started on July 2 and was getting worse every day. She asked the assistant if there was anything in her paperwork indicating that this was urgent and asked if she could be seen sooner. The assistant said no and then started reading out some of the information she had, including the radiologist's report, and mentioned the "severe edema of her lower limbs." Whoa! Lulu's problem had nothing to do with her limbs. Her limbs were not even included in her CT scan. Wrong CT report and wrong patient. Lulu asked her if the ER doctor had sent over the images and was told that she needed to bring them to the hospital in Hamilton herself. The assistant told her that if she wanted to be seen sooner, she could try to come in through emergency to get into the system, but there were no guarantees.

Things were not going well. Lulu picked up a CD of her CT images and headed to Hamilton to try to convince someone to take her spleen out. She waited for nine hours to see the surgeon on call. They scheduled a repeat ultrasound for the next morning and sent her home with a prescription for Tylenol 3 for the pain, only the pharmacy she went to couldn't fill the prescription because the doctor forgot to write his Ontario Medical Association number on the script. The pharmacist tried to call the hospital and get another script sent over, but nothing happened. Lulu waited until midnight, when the pharmacy closed, and then gave up and went home.

The next day, she had her second ultrasound. This again confirmed that she had a large and painful splenic mass. It was now 12 centimetres in diameter, which is impressive. The ER doctor had decided that Lulu would be best served by an infectious disease specialist. She thought that because Lulu was a veterinarian, it was possible/probable that this large splenic mass was an *Echinococcus* cyst, which is caused by a type of parasite. Veterinarians are more at risk for zoonotic diseases, but this was a bit of a leap. Most parasitic infections occur because of uncooked meat, poor hygiene, walking around barefoot in, say, India, and/or eating fecal material. Fecal–oral transmission is a concept that most veterinarians are fairly familiar with and try to avoid. But yes, Lulu had spent a lot of time with dogs, so an incredibly rare splenic *Echinococcus* cyst was now on the top of the list of potential causes of her splenic mass. An internal medicine resident came in to chat with her about her worms and she had a blood test for exposure to *Echinococcus*. She was sent home with prescriptions for Percocet (for pain) and expensive dewormers. She was told that someone would get in touch with her soon to book an appointment with the infectious disease specialist.

She returned the following week to the emergency room. The abdominal pain was increasing. Rather than moving toward actually treating the mass, the obvious next step was to do another ultrasound to document that she had a splenic mass. Her third abdominal ultrasound

revealed that the mass was in fact still there and still growing. There was a strong positive correlation between the
size of the mass and the amount of pain it was causing. At
this point, it was protruding from under her rib cage and
she could see it easily, not that she needed to, because she
was acutely aware of its existence through the pain, which
was now intolerable, and she could feel it swinging and
bobbing around in her abdomen as she walked.

It was July 30. She made it to her appointment with the
surgeon. The surgeon determined that she needed a splenectomy. Hallelujah! She signed consent forms for a splenectomy and cried in her surgeon's office because she was so
relieved to be making progress. The surgeon did not know
what was happening with her infectious disease specialist
appointment. He said that he would look into it. Someone would call her later in the week to give her a surgery
date and it would be very soon. He sent her home with a
prescription for hydromorphone tablets for pain, and his
office number. He told her to call if she needed anything.

Lulu tried to get in touch with the infectious disease
specialist to ask about her test results and/or an appointment, but was unsuccessful. She did finally manage to get
through to the emergency room, and by chance spoke to
the same internal medicine resident who had drawn blood
for her *Echinococcus* titres. She asked for the results and
the resident cheerfully told her, "They are negative, so you
are all cleared." The whole worm thing, previously considered to be her most likely diagnosis, now seemed to have
been dropped. No one ever addressed it again and she was
never contacted by the infectious disease specialist. She
ran out of pain medication and was unable to reach the

surgeon—the one who had told her to call if she needed anything. She headed into a long weekend without a refill or a surgery date. She was completely worn out.

On August 8, the surgeon's assistant called to tell her that they were booking her surgery for August 23. What? Why the delay? Well, because she did not have the required splenectomy vaccines, which need to be done fourteen days prior to the splenectomy, of course. She had been at the hospital talking to the surgeon nine days ago, signing the splenectomy consent form, and there was no mention of pre-splenectomy vaccines. (You can't make this shit up!) At this point, Lulu lost it. The assistant told her to call back once she had calmed down, and hung up on her.

She calmed down and phoned back. The assistant instructed her to go to her family doctor for her vaccinations, but Lulu didn't have a family doctor. She was also told that no one at the hospital could do the vaccines for her, which is hard to believe. She asked for a prescription for the vaccinations and for more pain medication, which was not possible to orchestrate until the next day. Once she finally had the vaccines in hand, I vaccinated Lulu because a physician was not available. I gave her the shots for pneumococcal pneumonia, *Haemophilus influenzae*, and *Meningococcus*. I waited with her for a while to make sure that she didn't have an anaphylactic reaction, filled out her vaccination record, and signed it with my name, followed by DVM. The countdown was on now—fourteen days until she could have her massive spleen removed. She was glad to have August 23 as her surgery date, but the chronic and worsening pain was taking its toll on her.

Meanwhile, at our veterinary teaching hospital, I met

a lovely German shepherd named Duke who came in through our oncology service. Duke is a good example of how veterinarians manage splenic masses. Duke arrived on August 16. He'd already had a sarcoma removed from his neck area on three separate occasions. It had never been removed with large margins, and microscopic amounts of cancer cells were left behind each time. Predictably, it recurred a few months after each surgery. Duke had a consultation with an oncologist, chest X-rays, and blood work performed all on the same day. The next day, he had a CT scan of his chest and the previous surgery site. We recommended an abdominal ultrasound, but it was declined by the owner for financial reasons. We discussed the CT results with the owner. There was no evidence that Duke's cancer had spread to his lungs, and we recommended surgery to take more tissue to try to prevent another recurrence.

Duke came back on August 22 to meet with me and be admitted for surgery. While we were getting ready for his surgery, my resident had a quick feel of Duke's abdomen. This had been impossible to accurately assess when Duke was awake because he was a big dog and his abdomen was tense, but now that he was under anesthetic and his abdomen was relaxed, we could feel an abdominal mass. My resident grabbed a portable ultrasound unit and took a look. Duke had a large, cavitated splenic mass. We ran down to radiology to see if we could get a full abdominal ultrasound, but all the appointments for the day were booked. We called the owner and recommended waking Duke up and doing a full abdominal ultrasound the next morning, just to make sure we knew what we were dealing with.

Duke came back the next day and had his ultrasound—
he had a 10-centimetre cavitated splenic mass. Everything
else in his abdomen looked normal. We contacted the
owner and he gave consent for us to do a splenectomy. His
mass could have been anything from a benign hematoma to
a very aggressive form of cancer called hemangiosarcoma.

So Duke took a short path and Lulu took a long and
arduous one. Duke and his owner had twenty-four hours
between the diagnosis of a splenic mass and a splenectomy, and Lulu had fifty-two days. By chance, both my
intern Lulu and my patient Duke were having their spleens
removed for large, cavitated splenic masses on August 23.
Duke was anesthetized and had a routine splenectomy by
an abdominal approach. He was in and out of surgery in
forty-five minutes. The spleen was submitted for histopathology. Duke recovered in our ICU overnight on pain
medication and intravenous fluids. He was eating, drink-
ing, walking, and comfortable the next day and he went
home that afternoon with his owner.

Lulu didn't have it quite so easy. The surgeons tried to
remove her spleen via laparoscopy, even though Lulu told
them she was fine with an open approach. This is a fantastic example of the perversion of intent. The intent of laparoscopy is to perform a surgical procedure through very
small incisions, to improve post-operative comfort and
healing and to decrease the length of the hospital stay. The
problem for Lulu was that her mass was 14 centimetres
at the last ultrasound, and it was growing and cystic. I'm
not sure that this scenario would ever lend itself to a small
incision. But a laparoscopic splenectomy is sexier and the
preferred technique in humans. The spleen is macerated

in a plastic bag within the abdomen and then pulled out through a small incision. Very slick, unless you have a huge, heavy mass and you are concerned about rupturing it. It makes handling, macerating, and putting it into a little bag a bit difficult.

Lulu was in surgery for four hours. The minimally invasive technique was attempted and failed. The surgeons had to convert to an open approach. She ended up with a 25-centimetre incision under her ribs on her left side. They had started with a smaller incision but had to extend it because the mass was so large and hard to handle. Her husband was in the waiting room the entire time and didn't receive any information about how her surgery was going until she was moved to recovery. He waited for over five hours with no news.

Minimally invasive techniques are truly a wonder, but they are not always all they are cracked up to be. They have side effects of their own. Having a failed laparoscopic splenectomy followed by an open splenectomy is like being in labour for twenty-four hours and then needing a C-section: it is the worst of both worlds. The gas used to inflate the abdomen for the laparoscopy is irritating to the abdominal lining, especially after a long procedure. It also hurts a lot when the gas moves around in the abdomen and when it moves out of the body, usually through the shoulders. On top of that, the 25-centimetre incision on her left side meant that she was agony when she woke up. She had traded her severe pain due to a splenic mass for severe pain due to surgery.

Lulu's spleen caused quite the stir. The surgeon came to see her and showed her photos on his iPhone of her ex-spleen and accompanying mass. He could not contain his excitement. The residents said it was the size of a basketball and was surprisingly heavy. Wow! I understand the enthusiasm. Physicians and veterinarians alike have a love for freaky medical anomalies, and I would probably be the same way if I had removed a spleen that size. (I have been). Lulu has a curious mind, and I think she could appreciate her fantastic splenic mass on some level, and the way the mass dwarfed her remaining normal spleen, and that it looked like a huge head (mass) with Mickey Mouse ears (spleen) on top of it. On the other hand, she had been through hell for the past seven weeks and it didn't seem to be getting much better. The cool pics were not helpful. She was hospitalized for five days while they tried to get her pain under control. She had some good nurses and some bad nurses, but overall, her stay in the hospital was horrible and she was miserable and in pain most of the time.

Meanwhile, Duke's histopathology came back and the splenic mass was a benign hematoma. This was not what I was expecting, but it was good news. Duke came back in two weeks and had the surgery he was originally scheduled to undergo before we found the splenic mass. He had the scar on his shoulder resected with bigger margins, with a goal of removing all of the cancer cells that might have been left behind. He went home the next day with oral pain medication. The histopathology report for the scar was available within a few days and his margins were tumour-free. Except for monitoring, Duke was done with his treatments.

Lulu removed her skin staples herself, eleven days after surgery. A few days later, she got a call from an elated pathology resident, which is unusual on many levels. Her mass was a benign congenital cyst, meaning it had existed from birth and was not cancer. They weren't sure why it suddenly grew, but it was good news. Usually, the surgeon would be the one to call with this news, but the pathology resident called Lulu because she wanted write up the case for publication. It is never a good thing to be a case report. Lulu acquiesced, but under one condition—she wanted to be included as an author on the article. After all, she was an integral part of her own medical team and she had her career to think about.

For Lulu, the huge relief of the benign diagnosis was overshadowed by the nightmare of her ordeal. Chronic pain, sleep deprivation, and the stress of waiting for a diagnosis do not discriminate between benign and malignant disease. For Duke, it was the opposite. His splenic mass was removed within a day of discovery; the biopsy report came back quickly with the good news that it was a benign hematoma. But eight months later, Duke returned to our hospital with metastatic cancer and was euthanized. On autopsy, he was confirmed to have widespread metastatic hemangiosarcoma, most likely from the initial splenic mass, which was, retrospectively, not benign. Ironically, if we'd had the correct diagnosis of hemangiosarcoma at the time and had treated him with chemotherapy and he had lived for eight months, we would have thought that was a huge success. We couldn't have cured him, and his owner was at least saved months of anguish thinking that his dog had a fatal form of cancer. Not that this was a good end to Duke's story. It was quite horrible and his owner was completely unprepared. The only silver lining was the lack of cancer dread. Cancer dread is inevitable, whether you have a diagnosis of cancer or you are waiting in the no man's land between surgery and the histopathology report.

Waiting for a histopathology report for yourself or your dog is hard. It creates a huge level of anxiety, and the only way to decrease that anxiety is to get the results back as quickly as possible and move on to the next steps. After my thyroid surgery, I found myself stuck in this purgatory. Waiting.

FOR THE FIRST TWO weeks after my surgery, I was so focused on recovering that I wasn't thinking about the histopathology results too much. I only started to get twitchy after three weeks. The angst escalated from there. I emailed my surgeon as directed, at the prescribed times, to remind him to look up my report. He emailed back his signature one-liner with instructions on when it would be appropriate for me to email him again with another reminder.

My surgeon told me that the report would take three weeks to come back after surgery. I found this astonishing; when it comes to my patients, I expect verbal reports of biopsy samples back within twenty-four hours, and a written report in forty-eight to seventy-two hours. If I don't get that level of service, I will contact the head of pathology and complain. I may be the only surgeon who requests histopathology samples to be run stat in certain cases. *Stat* is usually reserved for tests that you need immediately and that can be run on an emergency basis. Fixing tissues in formalin and then making slides to evaluate takes time, and there is no way to speed up this part of the process, so requesting a histopathology sample stat doesn't even make sense. I do it anyway. I know that I am being super-annoying, but I don't care, because I am an advocate for my patients and clients. Usually I do a biopsy to determine the diagnosis and then try to turn around the biopsy so that I can get the patient back in for definitive surgery within a week or two. I spend my on-clinics weeks in a state of adrenaline-fuelled panic, trying to crank the cases through. (There is just so much cancer out there.) This is partly because when it comes to cancer, faster treatment is better. But, for most cases, waiting a week or two is not going to make a difference to the outcome. The other part is that I don't want my clients to have to wait for their pet to have surgical treatment. Waiting is just too stressful. My patients, of course, are not too bothered by the waiting, as long as we keep them comfortable.

But me—I am stuck between the benign and the malignant. If you get a benign diagnosis, the stress and worry are supposed to instantly evaporate. It is not even a good story any more. You can't tell your friends about your other friend who triumphed over her benign cyst. No movies or books have been written to recount a tale of how someone overcame zero odds of losing and prevailed over a benign lump. We all get into the drama of pain and suffering—our own or someone else's. On some level, we love to tell people about the number of stitches we had; or the bone that was actually broken; or that it was pneumonia; or that it was *C. difficile*, not just a bad case of diarrhea; or that the big neck lump was cancer, not a cyst — it can be validating because it puts a name on our fear and proves that it's a big deal. People feel sorry for us and give us permission to feel sorry for ourselves. Then, if we don't feel sorry for ourselves, people think we are supertough. Heroes, even.

If it is just a cancer scare; or you're bruised and not broken; or your gash doesn't require stitches; or you only had a bad case of the flu, then you'd better pull yourself together and get back to work. You can't discuss the terrible anxiety you went through when you *thought* you had cancer. Where's the drama in that? No one will ever understand how hard that was and no one cares. They simply move on to the next horrific talking point. The best you can hope for is a few more sarcastic comments and jokes about how you let your knowledge and worry get the better of you. All the sleepless nights and stress deep within you were for nothing.

There is no web site for cancer fakers. I could try to start one — www.ialmosthadthyroidcancer.com — but it probably wouldn't get any sponsors, and no one would visit the site. Thyroid cancer fakers don't have ribbons, or stickers that look like ribbons, or magnets that look like stickers that look like ribbons. Fake thyroid tumours do not get an awareness month like real cancers. I'm not sure how you get a whole month for your cancer. With only twelve months to choose from and so many types of cancers, it's hard to fit all of the cancer into the year.

Every month seems to have multiple cancers and diseases assigned to it. Things start to get really busy in the fall. I guess the fall is the best time for conferences and cancer awareness because it works better for people with kids. It's competitive. September is bursting with hyper-awareness. It's cancer awareness month for childhood cancers, gynecologic cancer, Hodgkin's lymphoma, leukemia, lymphoma, melanoma, ovarian cancer, thyroid cancer, and prostate cancer. It's hard to be aware of so many cancers at the same time. I feel overstimulated and notice that I am becoming less aware. I have cancer awareness fatigue, which is another emerging syndrome. Breast cancer has taken October with no challengers. November, also a busy month, has five cancers to be aware of *and* it is Movember. Who doesn't like to see their bro grow a mo for cancer? So the super-lame mo has its renaissance every Movember to increase awareness of man cancers, but for some reason prostate cancer awareness month is in September.

Also wondering if an organ really needs a whole month. It's hard to keep track of all these organs getting cancer. Maybe we could organize our awareness by body system? Head, neck, and thyroid could share? Or maybe tobacco awareness should share with head and neck, or oral cancer, or maybe lung cancer? It's complicated. I'm disappointed that thyroid cancer gets mixed in with all of the other September cancers. Perhaps some of these cancers could drop back to just a week? A month is a long time to focus on only one cancer—just a suggestion. The whole thing seems really disorganized. Someone needs to take charge of the situation and come to a cancer awareness consensus. Like the European Union, but for cancer. Things get really quiet in December. I guess nobody wanted December for their cancer awareness month because people are too busy with the holidays. Christmas and cancer don't mix.

I feel a bit lost when it comes to the disease colour designations, too. There are so many ribbon colours. It's total chaos. Each one is supposed to be a symbol. A symbol, as in no words. If you have to write out the name of your cancer, disease, or cause on the ribbon because it is unrecognizable as a colour, then I think it's fair to say that your ribbon has failed to raise awareness. Some groups have tried to distinguish their ribbon with an unusual colour, such as periwinkle for bulimia and anorexia nervosa, but periwinkle has also been claimed by pulmonary hypertension. Who knew? Lime green is for Duchenne muscular dystrophy, regular muscular dystrophy, lymphoma, and Lyme disease. Lime green for Lyme disease is the only one that makes sense. Maybe muscular dystrophy and lymphoma should just back off and let Lyme disease have its own colour. Pearl is for lung cancer and a zebra-striped ribbon is for carcinoid cancer. I would argue that these aren't colours, but at least they are unique.

Pink and teal (together) signify thyroid cancer awareness. Pink on its own has been claimed by breast cancer, so no one else will touch pink with a ten-foot pole. You would think that teal would be relatively safe, but teal has also been claimed by post-traumatic stress disorder, rape, food allergies, ovarian cancer, polycystic ovarian syndrome, anti-bullying, and anxiety disorder. Why is teal so popular? It's bad enough that thyroid cancer has to borrow pink from the cancer superpower and we have to share September with so many other cancers because of Breast-tober, but now rape and thyroid cancer are both teal?

Then there are the T-shirts, bracelets, stickers, and swag to display your awareness. Some cancers even have animals. There is no animal to symbolize the benign thyroid mass, but thyroid cancer gets a butterfly because the shape of a normal thyroid gland looks like a bowtie or a butterfly. What could be more beautiful and symbolic than a butterfly to represent your cancer metamorphosis? You break out of your cocoon of darkness and float around in the September sun. Benign? No butterfly for you. Also, if you don't have cancer, you can just forget about wearing any paraphernalia that says things like "Fight Like a Girl" or "Cancer Chicks" or "Fuck Cancer." Not for you; you're just not that tough. You don't even have cancer, remember?

The thyroid cancer surgery scar is an awareness campaign in itself. I keep imagining crossing paths with another woman who has the same scar. First we glance over each other's neck scars and then our eyes meet—we nod and point our left hands down low in a slow, cool recognition of our oneness, like two bikers on Harleys meeting on a highway. Only, if all you had was a benign cyst or thyroiditis, it would be a total sham. You're not tough at all. The two women comparing scars would be sisters until it came out that one of them just had a...cyst. It doesn't matter that they both had a mass and surgery and thought for months that they might have cancer. They are not the same.

Cancer fakers can't use words like *remission, monitoring, radioactive iodine, metastasis,* or *survival time.* Those words do not belong to them. Benign. Done. Never coming back. Cured, but not through groundbreaking medical innovation and cancer research, or the positive attitude of a cancer warrior princess, or the tenacity of the human spirit, but because the disease was impotent, weak, and ineffective. So ineffective that this pathetic collection of cells can't even call itself cancer. Technically, even a benign growth could be called cancer by a very loose definition, but what really separates the benign from the malignant is whether or not the cells are immortal. Normal cells have controls that tell them how much to grow, when to reproduce and, most important, when to die. Cancer cells continue to live, grow, and divide beyond any of our innate controls or signals. They are permanently turned on and they don't listen to the rest of the body. If the cells are immortal then we are not, and that is cancer.

FROM THE MOMENT I first felt the mass in my neck, I knew it was a thyroid carcinoma. I can't explain why; I just did. Unfortunately, I was the only one who felt this way. Four physicians, with differing levels of certainty, told me I was wrong. So did many of my friends and colleagues. Perhaps it was because benign disease is so much more common, or because my hysteria was mistaken for hypochondria, or maybe it was because nobody wants to think that their friend, colleague, or patient has cancer, but the conflict between the internal and external voices left me feeling crazy.

As a veterinary surgeon, I have come to rely on a few things. The first is my fingers. They are well-trained. I trust them to receive and transmit a lot of information, both when I am examining a patient and when I am in surgery. I suspect they are more sensitive than other people's fingers. When I say that this mass is new and it wasn't there two days before I found it, I am 100 percent sure because my fingers are 100 percent sure.

Then there is my brain. I am not a genius, but I am smart. I have worked hard to understand medicine and at least a small part of how cancer works. Early recognition and treatment are a good start in the fight against cancer. Taking a "wait and see" approach to a fast-growing mass is contrary to everything that I know about cancer.

Next is my intuition. Almost every mistake I have ever made as a veterinarian was because I didn't listen to my gut. Sometimes the medical decisions I make are because of feeling something rather than thinking it through. It is taking one look at a patient and knowing that he is going to live or die, and being sure. I have come to define myself through my fingers, brain, and intuition, and now everyone is telling me that everything I know and trust is wrong.

The self-doubt creeps in. How can it not? I am so sure that I am right, but someone is wrong—either all these doctors or me. Maybe I am just freaking out and thinking it is cancer because I work with cancer. I know that's what everybody thinks. Some people have determined I am nuts because I dropped everything when I found this mass and started demanding immediate medical attention for something that will likely turn out to be nothing. Maybe I secretly want to have cancer (although I have no idea why anyone would, but maybe this is what happens to people who work too much and then crack up); maybe that is why I keep insisting (if only to myself and occasionally to my husband, because I am too embarrassed to say it to anyone else) it is going to be a carcinoma. Given the choice between losing my mind and cancer, which do I choose?

Maybe this ridiculous melodrama is just a plea for attention from an overworked, burnt-out dog cancer doctor. Maybe I am just a big fat cancer faker.

Adding to this anxiety, I am now back at work and people are asking about my diagnosis. They ask me when I see them in the bathroom or walking down the hall, as I am scrubbing in to surgery, when I am doing surgery, and as I am sitting down to a meeting. Always in public spaces, and always when there is no time or space to talk about cancer.

In some ways, it is good that I don't have any news yet. How am I supposed to respond to the person who is simultaneously passing me in the hall, eating lunch, texting, and walking a dog as they quickly look up and say, "Hey, Sarah, how's it going? Got your histo back yet?" Should I just keep walking and say, "Yeah, it's cancer, thanks for checking, see ya later"? Who's the asshole here? The person asking or the person dropping the C-bomb? I know it is because they care, or maybe it's because they are curious, or chatty, or socially inept, but it's a good lesson: don't ask a question if you are not prepared for a negative answer. My first thought was that this is because people are basically insensitive and stupid, but reflecting further I think it is because, as a group, we like to gawk at car accidents. We like to get close enough to touch, but not close enough for a direct hit. There is some solid entertainment value in cancer. Talking about our friends with cancer gives us some authority. We have seen some things; we know a thing or two about life. It's cancer porn.

When I try to see this curious behaviour in a more positive light, I come up with this: maybe it is human nature to look for the positive outcome. We have answered the question before it comes out of our mouths. We are asking because we hope everything is okay, not because we imagine that the person we are asking is experiencing the worst-case scenario. We expect the fine and not the awful; the perfect happy baby and not the miscarriage; the benign and not the malignant; the cure and not the death. We should know better by now. Life doesn't always work out that way.

ONE NIGHT WHEN MY guard is down, I miss a call from my surgeon because I am on the phone with my mom discussing why I have not heard about my results yet, despite four weeks having passed.

I check the message, which is more telling in what is left out than what is said. "Hi, Sarah, it's Adam. (*Pause.*) I will try to call you tomorrow." The results are conspicuous in their absence and I know this is not good. I have left the same message for clients myself. When I have bad news for a client, I can't leave it on the answering machine. In this case, no news is bad news and I know it. The call is blocked and he doesn't leave a number to call him back at and it's late. I have done that too. I send him a sad little email about how sorry I am to have missed his call, and even though he will get the message instantly, I know that the window has closed for the night. This message confirms the feeling in my heart that I have a carcinoma, but I can't talk about it to anyone because it will just fuel the ever-growing case that I have lost my mind if this does turn out to be benign disease. I keep it to myself for one more day.

My surgeon reaches me the next day, almost a full twenty-four hours later. I have been at an all-day seminar for work and am sitting next to the door in case I have to leave to answer the phone. My cellphone has been in my hand for most of the day, and I have been obsessively checking it every five minutes, just in case I missed a call. Then, with the phone in my pocket and on vibrate, I miss the call. How is that even possible? It goes to voicemail as I panic and race out of the room. Mercifully, he has left a number this time so I can call him back and I am able to reach him. He tells me that my mass has come back as a papillary thyroid carcinoma. I was right: I have thyroid cancer. He finds this a bit surprising (I do not) because my cytology results from the initial needle biopsy were benign (actually they weren't), so he has contacted the pathologist and discussed the results with him and has asked for a second pathologist to evaluate my histopathology to confirm the results. The first pathologist is sure about this being cancer. I tell him that the cytology results were non-diagnostic, not benign. I can hear him typing on the computer as he looks up my non-diagnostic cytology results and agrees that it makes a lot more sense now.

When he has finished typing, we talk about a plan. The second pathologist still has to confirm this diagnosis (or maybe it's not needed now—hard to tell), which will take another two weeks (wow!). If it is confirmed, I will have to have a second surgery to remove the rest of my thyroid gland. This is the first week since my surgery that I have started to feel like myself, and the thought of having to go through it all again is more than a little disappointing. He had talked about a second surgery to remove the rest of my thyroid gland as a remote possibility during my initial appointment. He said that if the results came back as a carcinoma, the second surgery would be in two to three months. I am not sure what this timeline means, though. It's confusing. Two to three months from my first surgery? Two to three months from this phone call? Two to three months from the second pathologist's report? Or two to three months from our next appointment, which is going to be a week or two after the second pathologist's report? The bottom line is that it is a carcinoma and I need more surgery and it will be some time in the next one to four months.

There is some good news in this call. The surgical margins are clean and there is no vascular invasion, which means that he excised it all; the cancer cells do not seem to be heading into the blood vessels or lymphatic vessels, which is how they metastasize to other locations. I ask him whether or not I will need radioactive iodine treatment and he says we won't decide that right now, but he thinks it is unlikely. The formula used to decide is based on the tumour size, the pathologist's report, blood levels of thyroglobulin, and whether or not it has metastasized to the lymph nodes. (Mine have not been biopsied, but I don't ask about this again.) He says I am in a low-risk group for needing radioactive iodine because the mass was only 2.7 centimetres. I try not to be too cheeky and annoying but I correct him again and say that it may not make a difference, but the mass was actually 3.7 to 3.8 centimetres. There is more tapping while he looks at my report again. He tells me that the pathology report says the mass was 3.2 centimetres and the size on the pathology report is what they use to make recommendations about radioactive iodine treatment. I start to worry about whether they looked at the size of the mass before or after it went into formalin, because tissues shrink after they are fixed in formalin. From what I have read, there doesn't seem to be a consensus on the size cut-off for recommending radioactive iodine, or if this measurement is based on ultrasound or on the mass itself, before or after it is placed in formalin. He is obviously not concerned about it today and we have finished talking now. I thank him and get off the phone.

I am in shock with this not-shocking news. I am feeling a lot of things, but one dominant feeling is relief. *Relief* is not the best word, but there is no better word for my reaction. I am relieved by bad news. I am mal-relieved. The shoe dropped; the waiting is over. I am mal-relieved that the internal and external dialogues are now consistent with one another. I am mal-relieved that my gut instincts were correct. I am mal-relieved that I listened to myself, and I am mal-relieved that things can move forward. I am not a hypochondriac. I am not a cancer faker.

Despite the heavy news, there are two things that make me feel a bit lighter today. The mass is out and it seems that it has been completely removed, and the struggle is over. Not the struggle with the disease, but the fight to be heard. This cancer chick did have to fight like a girl, but it was the system I was fighting, more than the disease. I was fighting to get treatment and to keep listening to myself. Cancer is still a worthy opponent; I know that. But compared to what is behind me, I can definitely handle a little touch of cancer.

IF YOU ARE A dog with a mass or a lump that someone thinks is cancer, your path to diagnosis and treatment will be very different than mine, with one glaringly obvious similarity: every patient needs an advocate. This is probably more apparent in canine patients because they can't discuss their clinical signs, take themselves to the doctor, or make any decisions about their health. They are completely reliant on health advocacy.

As a dog, your fate will depend on several factors, none of which you will have any control over or could possibly understand. The first factor is whether or not your family veterinarian thinks you have cancer. This could be good or bad for you. If your family veterinarian thinks you have cancer, but also has a personal belief that most cancers in animals are not treatable and that dogs do not do well with aggressive cancer treatment, the spin they put on your presumptive diagnosis will not be good. In these cases, only the most persistent clients will reject the idea that their dog is old and probably has bad cancer and the most sensible and humane thing to do would be to let them go—and soon. If your vet thinks you have cancer, and gets on it quickly with a good diagnostic plan and a referral to a specialist to discuss the options, you have a chance. If your vet missed the fact that you might have cancer altogether, then precious time will have been wasted on symptomatic treatments that will not improve your situation.

The second factor is your owner. Did they notice that something was wrong with you and take you to a doctor in the first place?

Money is also a major factor. All the tests and procedures cost money. Your veterinarian needs to know what to recommend and how to explain the value of these tests to your owner. Your owner needs to understand the recommendations, and want to move forward, and be able to afford the care. Where you fit into your household is also important. Are you a four-legged, furry child? Do you sleep in the same bed as your owner? If you have never achieved this status, or if you have lost it because of the appearance of real, two-legged, fur-less children, things may not go well for you. Your owner's opinion of cancer and previous experiences with this disease will also play a role. Many clients will say, "If it's cancer, I don't want to treat," or "If it's cancer, there is nothing we can do about it anyway," not realizing that some cancers are more treatable than many chronic health problems. If you are a dog, your whole life hangs in the balance of perception.

SADIE WAS A FOUR-YEAR-OLD Australian shepherd who came to see me when I was working as a small animal surgeon in western Canada. Her owner was a single guy in his late twenties. He was very outdoorsy and he and his dog were a great match. They were the type of dog–owner combo you would expect to see in a Fido commercial. They were both young, active, intelligent, attractive, and a bit rugged. On one of her outdoor adventures, Sadie developed a cough and was taken to her family veterinarian. X-rays of her chest showed a large mass in her lung. It looked like lung cancer. The owner said that he was told he should feed her lots of steaks because she was going to die soon, and this was the only treatment option discussed. Steak. I guess, for some, feeding lots of steaks is the doggie equivalent of the Make-A-Wish Foundation, but it is not a treatment and it is not very doctor-y to tell this to a client. You do not get out your prescription pad and write (illegibly) *1 x steak, rare, by mouth once daily x 14 days (or until death)*, and then send your client to the local grocer to fill it. Lung cancer in dogs is treatable with surgery and chemotherapy; patients can achieve long-term remission and even be cured in some cases.

Sadie's owner was devoted to her and her greatest advocate. He was unsatisfied with both the diagnosis and the treatment plan and went straight to the Internet to try to solve her problem. Normally, clients who do this come up with some crazy and cringeworthy theories, but his research was sound. He and Sadie had spent time camping and hiking in southern Saskatchewan, which is endemic for blastomycosis, a systemic fungal infection. The owner determined that his dog did not have cancer, but a fungal

infection in her lungs that required a prescription for ketoconazole (an antifungal medication). He told me his theory
during our consultation. I was amused. He had lost faith
in veterinarians and was going it alone. His only reason
for coming to see me was to trade his steak prescription for
a ketoconazole prescription.

I took a look at Sadie's X-rays, which were a few weeks
old. There was a solitary mass in the lung that did look like
it could be a tumour, but it could be something else too,
with a fungal infection on the list. I recommended that we
do some blood tests to see how she was doing systemically, as well as repeat the X-rays of her lungs to see what
they looked like now. He resisted. He didn't see the point
when he knew in his heart that his dog had blastomycosis.
I explained to him that the drugs he wanted for her were
extremely expensive, needed to be given for months, and
had a lot of potential side effects, so a diagnosis was essential before I could start her on them.

Sadie's new X-rays showed diffuse lung disease with
a pattern that was much more consistent with a fungal
infection. We did a transtracheal wash, which requires
the patient to be sedated while a sterile sample of cells,
fluid, and accompanying goo from the trachea and lungs
is aspirated into a syringe. She was stoic and tolerant of
us during this somewhat barbaric procedure. We got a lot
of goo back, which was great because it meant we were
more likely to get a diagnosis. We examined the material
under the microscope; it told us everything we needed to
know. There were reams and reams of fungal hyphae in
the sample, meaning that we could see fungus actively
growing in her lungs. We still sent the material away for

a pathologist to confirm. The pathologist agreed it was blastomycosis.

I told the owner the results. He gave me a look that said, "I told you so." I returned a look that said, "I never said it wasn't." Sadie started her medication. She didn't have cancer, which was wonderful, but a systemic fungal infection is no picnic either. It is hard to treat and takes months of expensive medications and recheck examinations. Like cancer, it can recur, but at least it is curable. Sadie's infection spread to her bones during her treatment course, and the treatment was hard on her, but she recovered fully.

I started out as an antifungal medication prescription vehicle but turned into a partner in getting Sadie healthy again. The owner was so happy about everything I actually started to worry that he had developed the classic client-to-vet crush. Superawkward. This happens from time to time with veterinarians and clients. It has a lot less to do with who we are than with what we give to our clients. We listen to them and give them our time and attention. We also give them hope and unconditional love. Not our own, but the unconditional love of their dog is returned to them, at least for some time. If you can give someone hope and unconditional love, you are not just crush-worthy, you are a religion. You are Jesus in a white coat. I moved away and left this owner with his one true love, Sadie, now healthy and ready for more outdoor adventures.

Mike was another lung cancer faker that I treated. (Side thought: I love when people give their pets regular people names, like Mike and Sadie.) Mike was a three-and-a-half-year-old male Labrador retriever. Mike had everything going for him. He was the proverbial perfect nuclear family pet. He was handsome, active, smart, well-behaved, and protective of his family. He was great with the kids and he loved his dad most of all. He was one of those dogs who seems to know what everyone wants from him and he obliged without being asked or trained. Until now, he had been the picture of health. He and his entire family looked like they had just walked out of the pages of an L. L. Bean catalogue: a beautiful, happy professional couple with a few gorgeous kids, a large disposable income, and a gorgeous designer dog. Like Sadie, Mike developed a cough and had X-rays done of his chest. He also had a large, solitary lung mass that looked very suspicious for cancer. Instead of interpreting this finding as a terminal event, Mike's veterinarian referred him to our oncology service for further workup and to discuss treatment options.

Mike's owner told us to do whatever we needed to do. He was not fazed by the potential cancer diagnosis or the quote. Mike had a CT scan, and we could see that one lobe of his lung was completely consolidated but no other areas were affected. The two most likely diagnoses were cancer or a parasitic disease. He was negative for the parasitic disease on a fecal test, but this test can result in false negatives, meaning that the test is negative but the patient has the disease. Either way, this lung lobe had been destroyed by either infection or cancer and it needed to be removed. The owner consented. We took Mike to surgery for a lung lobectomy. After surgery, I cut into the affected lobe; the multiple cystic areas in the lung were consistent with parasitic disease. I was so excited for Mike and his family that I could barely contain myself. I was so relieved that his owner had been willing to treat, despite the potential for bad news. Mike was young, strong, and otherwise healthy, and he recovered well. He went home two days later with pain medications and instructions to rest. At discharge, Mike ran out the door and did not look like he planned on resting much. The results came back and confirmed the good news. He had a parasitic infection called *Paragonimus*, not cancer. Mike and his beautiful family never looked back.

A dog with a cough and a lung mass can be spun as a death sentence or a treatable health problem, depending on how you approach it and on the underlying cause. Not every lung mass is cancer, even if things look bad. Not every case of lung cancer is fatal. An owner who is a strong advocate and who has the financial wherewithal can navigate past the barriers to get to a diagnosis and hopefully a resolution. But not every dog is so lucky. Sometimes the barriers to a diagnosis and treatment are too great and our patients lose before they even have the chance to fight. Sometimes just the word *cancer*, and not the disease itself, is enough to bring a dog's life to an end, even if it is a suggestion and not a firm diagnosis. A dog's life is only as important as we think it is, and it is only worth as much as we can afford, or choose, to pay. A dog's death is only as sad as it makes the owners who loved him, and a dog's recovery from cancer or fake cancer is only as happy as it makes the people who are cheering him on.

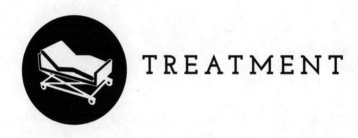

TREATMENT

I AM ABSORBING THE news of my diagnosis—at a spa. I am sitting in an outdoor hot tub at one of those Scandinavian therapeutic water circuits. It's the kind where you rotate between various pools of different temperatures, steam rooms, and wood-fired saunas. It is a science. You go from hot to cold (no thanks, I like it hot!) to the relaxation rooms. It is detoxifying and oh so relaxing. The brochure you receive when you check in is intended to make sure you relax properly and at the appropriate temperatures. Hot, cold, relax, repeat. Accompanying the heating and cooling pools are signs with a cartoon figure that is shushing everyone aggressively, reminding them that this is a place of "enforced silence." I realize that some people may not appreciate the silence. I read a few pretty ticked-off reviews on TripAdvisor from a few rowdy chicks who were unceremoniously shushed by the real and cartoon people here.

I, on the other hand, am all about the enforced silence. The quieter, the better. I need peace right now, and the last thing I want is some Bridezilla and her gang of heinous bridesmaids squawking about nails, hair, napkin colours, wedding dresses, bridesmaids' dresses, flowers, shower, stagette, strippers, lingerie, guest list, seating arrangement drama, potential bridesmaid-groomsmen hookups, or any of the thrilling twists and turns leading up to her stupid fucking perfect special day. No. You will need to take that rowdy fun elsewhere. You don't get to take over this space. This place is Zen, and right now, it's mine. There are people walking around in fluffy robes in various stages of heat stroke. No one is talking because they either want the quiet or have been shushed or ejected. The place feels like rehab, and for me, it is a sort of rehab: cancer rehab.

I take a break from my newly established hot tub, steam room, sauna cycle for a much-needed massage. I am filling out my health questionnaire before my treatment. It starts out with the basics: Name; Age; Sex; Have you had a massage before? Where does it hurt? Then it delves deep into my medical history. Although the questionnaire is for a relaxation massage at a spa, it asks for a more complete medical history than all of the forms I have filled out for my GP, endocrinologist, pre-operative nurse, anesthesiologist, and head-and-neck surgeon combined. I fill out the checklist:

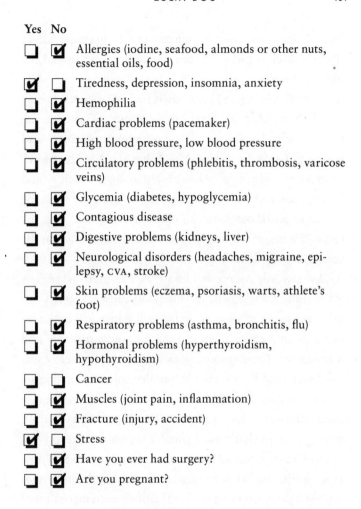

Yes No

☐ ☑ Allergies (iodine, seafood, almonds or other nuts, essential oils, food)

☑ ☐ Tiredness, depression, insomnia, anxiety

☐ ☑ Hemophilia

☐ ☑ Cardiac problems (pacemaker)

☐ ☑ High blood pressure, low blood pressure

☐ ☑ Circulatory problems (phlebitis, thrombosis, varicose veins)

☐ ☑ Glycemia (diabetes, hypoglycemia)

☐ ☑ Contagious disease

☐ ☑ Digestive problems (kidneys, liver)

☐ ☑ Neurological disorders (headaches, migraine, epilepsy, CVA, stroke)

☐ ☑ Skin problems (eczema, psoriasis, warts, athlete's foot)

☐ ☑ Respiratory problems (asthma, bronchitis, flu)

☐ ☑ Hormonal problems (hyperthyroidism, hypothyroidism)

☐ ☐ Cancer

☐ ☑ Muscles (joint pain, inflammation)

☐ ☑ Fracture (injury, accident)

☑ ☐ Stress

☐ ☑ Have you ever had surgery?

☐ ☑ Are you pregnant?

The cancer question tripped me up, now that I am a person who has to check this box. Cancer is a bit too big for a check box. I look up from my questionnaire. My massage therapist is here to collect me. She looks at my scar and then at my form. She is all over it. Once we are in the privacy of my massage room, I tell her that I recently had surgery to remove my right thyroid and that I have thyroid cancer. She then tells me that cancer and massage "don't really go well together" because massage can "spread the toxins." I am not sure what this means, but I haven't slept since my diagnosis and my body is tied up in knots. I tense up, thinking that she is going to refuse to massage me because of the well-known incompatibility of cancer and massage. I wonder if she thinks that she has the power to make my cancer worse with a massage, which would be impressive. All I was hoping for was someone with the power to work out these knots in my back and help me relax. We negotiate. She is concerned about spreading the cancer, energy flow, toxins, and lymphatics.

As a word, *toxins* is almost as overused as *cancer*. To be fair, some toxins definitely do cause cancer. Constant exposure to certain toxins will damage the DNA in our cells and cause them to replicate uncontrollably and metastasize. There is some weak evidence that a heavy seafood diet may be a factor in the development of thyroid cancer, due to the high iodine content. I have not eaten meat for twenty-four years but have been a pescetarian during most of that time. I wonder how many shrimp and other bottom-feeders I have consumed in my life and how much iodine was concentrated in their little shrimpy bodies. Should I stop eating seafood? Does it even matter now?

I am also wondering about continuing to use a lead thyroid collar at work. When we take X-rays of our patients, we wear a lead gown and a lead collar to protect us from the radiation. The lead collar is worn specifically to protect the thyroid gland from harmful X-rays that may cause thyroid cancer with enough exposure. I have always been religious/neurotic about wearing lead at work. I am glad about it now because at least I can't look back and think that I caused my thyroid cancer by being lax about radiation safety. Nope, I am definitely too much of a geek for that. Is there any point in wearing the collar now? I won't have a thyroid soon, so maybe not. Is it like a smoker who keeps smoking through lung or throat cancer treatment? You know, the guy in the anti-smoking commercial who is inhaling and exhaling smoke through his neck hole? Is the horse already out of the barn? One notable exception is that I hope to be a long-term cancer survivor with this milder form of cancer, much luckier than those with most smoking-related cancers, so maybe I do need to lay off the shrimp and keep up with the lead.

I convince my masseuse that I am not here for a cancer-curing massage, just relaxation, and tell her she can steer clear of my scary thyroid area if she is worried about the obvious dangerous effects of massage in this region. I nod as she tells me about how excessive stimulation of this area could be *very* detrimental to my recovery. She is clearly very worried about exacerbating my cancer with her bare hands, but she concedes, and gives me a great massage. I am relaxed for the first time in months. After the massage, I head back to the pools and steam room for more extreme heat and silence. I spend four hours there. I can't get enough.

I can't get enough of anything that will allow me to relax and/or take my mind off the diagnosis and the waves of emotions that go with it. A friend of mine emailed me that she was sorry to hear about my cancer scare. But it isn't a cancer scare when you actually have cancer. A cancer scare is when you think you have cancer and it turns

out that you don't. It's scary, but you can go back to normal. You will probably quickly forget all the things that
you thought you would change during your cancer scare:
the people you would be nicer to, the time you would take
off work, the way you would live life to the fullest. When
you are dealing with the cancer and not the scare, you
need to find a new way to live without being scared all the
time. You need to find your new normal.

Waves of fear wash over me, but they are more fear of
what just happened and how it could have turned out than
fear of the present. I think of how badly things could have
turned out if I had not had medical training and pushed
for surgery, if I had listened to the doctors who told me
that I should just "wait and see" and that I "didn't have
cancer" and that the mass was almost certainly "benign."
I feel the way you feel when you narrowly escape a really
bad car accident. You are so freaked out by the near miss
that you have to pull over and calm yourself down. That
is what I am attempting to do now. I'm pulling off the
highway, putting on my hazard lights, and trying to calm
myself down before I start driving again.

Cancer has definitely made me appreciate the important things in life, like Visa. My credit card has taken a
beating during the past few months. I just throw down
the C-card and all purchases are forgiven. Every day is
like my birthday, and then, on my actual birthday, which
coincided with the week I found out that this cancer scare
was for real, my husband surprised me with a brand-new
shiny red Vespa. Now that I have cancer, I can shop indis-
criminately: I recently bought many scarves to hide my
hideous neck scar, new clothes to go with the new scarves,

a MacBook Air, a new iPhone, and sparkly high-heeled shoes (I can't walk in them and have nowhere to wear them). There is no retribution or judgement, except in the form of a fat Visa bill and crippling interest rates. You can lay low from work, ignore gossip and your emails, miss deadlines, and generally let things slide, and it's all okay.

I am trying to put on a brave face for my friends. I am not sure if I am going to be an inspiring cancer patient or not. I sent out a cute group email, accompanied by a picture of me with my new Vespa:

Subject: news about my thyroid

Hi all,

Sorry for the group email. I wanted to let you know that I got my histo back today. So a bit of bad news: turns out it was a papillary carcinoma and I have to have my left thyroid out in a few months.

Good news:

1. The margins are clean and there are no characteristics of vascular/lymphatic invasion. ☺

2. This type of cancer is curable with my favourite cancer treatment: surgery. ☺

3. I was right. I know you are all amazed at the lengths that I will go just to be right. Yes, I really am that stubborn. ☺

4.   I now have major street cred. 😎

Thanks everyone for being so supportive. I am super-
lucky to have you in my life.

Attached picture is the surprise new Vespa that Steve got
me for my birthday!!! Excellent distraction and, yes, pretty,
shiny things do make me happy: today and every day.

Love,
Sarah

Maybe I overdid it. Maybe all those happy faces accompanying each line were a bit too much, because most of
the people replying seem to think that this news is simply
fantastic! Yes, I had cancer, but the mass is out and I got
a new Vespa, so I am good to go! I'm glad that everyone
thinks I am okay and am putting on a brave emoticon.
Then I start to feel sad and realize that I don't know how I
am supposed to act right now. I feel like I need a good cry
but I can't get the tears out. I need sleep but I have insomnia. It's as though I am trapped in a bad eighties power
ballad that I can't turn off. I'm so emotional.

Next stop on the cancer rehab train—a trip to the Caymans to teach at an offshore veterinary school. I didn't
plan to be in the Caymans while dealing with this news,
but cancer is much easier to take in the Caribbean. Pretty
much everything is easier to deal with there. I actually forgot about the whole thing a few times as I sat on the seven-
mile-long white sand beach and looked out at the beautiful
Caribbean Sea.

Grand Cayman is the main island of the Caymans. Even with a name like Grand, it is pretty small and has no fresh water. Almost everything gets imported into the country, even the tropical fruit. All the water comes from a desalinator, which is run by coal power. There is no recycling, just an overcrowded dump that takes up a fair percentage of the land mass. During the last major hurricane, the entire island was completely submerged and was lost to radar contact. If global warming continues at its current pace and sea levels keep rising, I imagine that this island will be gone in a few decades. I am amazed by the lack of eco-awareness, except in the odd billboard promoting "eco-chic," which is just faux environmentalism.

What is wrong with these people? Can't they see that they are on an island? Why don't they treat their environment with more respect? They are going to use up all of the resources here and then it will be too late. Then I realize that we are all on an island; it is just that some of us are on massive islands we call continents. The overcrowding is just as real and our supply of resources is just as limited. We are destroying our islands just as aggressively as the people on Grand Cayman, but we live as though the land, water, and energy will last forever.

This is what cancer does: it shows you that you are an island. It shows you that although you thought your life was going to go on forever, it has boundaries and one day it will be gone. The resources that we take for granted, namely our health and our life, are finite, but we don't see it because there is too much life stretched out all around us. We can't imagine ever making it to the edge. Cancer shows us that, one day, we will submit to our own ecological crisis. The toxins, our lifestyle, our bad genes, bad luck, or the years will catch up with us and we will be completely submerged, off the radar screen forever. You can try to slow the effects of global warming and carcinogenesis and grapple for a cure, but ultimately, whether this cancer is going to take you or not, life is short. Cancer sends us this message. Take care of yourself and enjoy your time here. You have now entered the real-life phase of your life.

I return from the Caymans and am thrust back into the reality of home, work, and cancer. I have an appointment with the endocrinologist who told me twice that I didn't have cancer and reported my cytology results to me inaccurately as benign. I am hoping he can help me overcome my sloth-like behaviour with an increased dose of thyroid medication. Waves of anger hit me when I think about meeting with him. I am mad as hell. I am planning on showing him just how angry I am as part of my cancer rehab. I want to tell him that whatever his motives were for telling me this mass was benign, it made it so much worse for me emotionally. I want to try to ensure that he doesn't do this to anyone again. Some people have suggested that I complain to the College of Physicians and Surgeons about his behaviour or sue him. I am not sure what that would accomplish and all I really want is an apology.

I am a bit jacked up when I arrive at my appointment. My doctor comes in, sits down, and starts reading my file. The blood and his good mood drain from his face. He is reading my histopathology report for the first time. He tells me that he is shocked and surprised that my thyroid mass has been diagnosed as a papillary thyroid carcinoma. He expresses his surprise a few more times and shows me

notes in my file where he wrote that he thought I had goit-
erous thyroiditis (benign inflammation of the thyroid). He
shakes his head, and then he shakes my hand and says
that he is so glad they did the right thing for me. He is so
sincere and so nice. The angry speech I had prepared in my
head evaporates. What am I supposed to say now? "I have
cancer, so there?"

Maybe it is not the worst thing in the world to have
an endocrinologist who is a bit humbled by his patient.
At least now he might listen to me when I tell him that
I don't feel right and need some adjustments to my dose,
and that I don't want to get fat or have bad hair. I know he
was doing what he thought was best, and he seemed to be
blindsided by this diagnosis.

My endocrinologist and I keep talking. He tells me
again he is shocked. I tell him that I am not shocked at
all. He tells me that it was very serendipitous that I had
surgery, and I suspect he does not know what this word
means because it was far from serendipitous. That would
suggest it had been left to chance. Nothing in medicine can
be left to serendipity. But I can't be mad at someone who is
so genuine and so kind. It is a cliché coming from someone
who has just been diagnosed with cancer, but I am not
sure how these negative emotions are going to serve me. I
wish I could say that since I was diagnosed, I have found
inner peace because I realized that I am an island, but I
don't always feel so peaceful.

At this moment, *manic* would be a better word for how
I feel. I still have some time left this summer before my
second surgery. I race around, working and playing hard
and travelling when I can. I'm trying to make the most

of it before the next phase of treatment begins. The more stimulated and distracted, the better. I know that it is all going to catch up with me at some point. You can't outrun the stages of cancer grief forever, but for now I am going to keep moving as fast as I can.

THINGS COULD ALWAYS BE worse! This is a well-intentioned but ridiculous thing to say to someone going through bad times. I have heard it a lot lately. My cancer is a good cancer, so yes, things could absolutely be worse. It could have spread to my lymph nodes, and that would be worse. Or my husband could take all of our money and run away with a twenty-five-year-old receptionist with big boobs, leaving me penniless, homeless, self-consciously flat-chested, and alone with my good cancer. Definitely worse. Or he could take my cat, too. Now, that would be unthinkable. At what point is it bad enough that it cannot get much worse? Or at least that people stop saying that? How bad does it have to get before people stop with the upbeat, preachy reminders? I think that is when you know that what is happening to you is truly awful, when you cross over the threshold of positive chatter into the silence that surrounds you when no one knows quite what to say. I don't always know the best thing to say either, but I have been struck by the power of receiving a card that simply says, "Thinking of you," or a friend who says, "How can I help?" The times when you don't know what to say are usually the times when your friends and family need to hear from you the most.

Along with the endless need for people to point out how happy we should be about the sort of bad—but not horrific—things that are happening to us, there is also the human need to rationalize these events, as if the universe is orchestrating all of the shit to be fertilizer in the garden of life. This sentiment is usually presented with the same sing-songy, up talking voice saying, "You see, everything happens for a reason!" (Some people have even suggested that getting thyroid cancer was really a lucky break because it gave me the opportunity to write a book. So not only did I get good, curable cancer but it resulted in becoming a published author. Lucky me!) Part of this rationale seems to underestimate the individual's role in overcoming adversity, like she/he has no control of the situation. (In my case it would be, "The universe gave you cancer and then the universe treated your cancer and made you an author, which will all be worth it if you get to meet Oprah or Ellen—or both—and it was all part of the grand plan that the universe had for you.") Sometimes I think "shit happens" is the most prophetic thing I have ever heard.

I am not sure what the universe is thinking sometimes. The universe can really kick the shit out of people. I am not talking about myself. I put my thyroid cancer in the moderately bad category. When it's all said and done, I will continue to live my charmed life among the lucky people until the next moderately bad thing happens. But the universe can be cruel. If I am seeing a client about their pet, then they already have one problem—their dog probably has cancer. But sometimes that is just the icing on the shitty cake and there is a long list of moderately to horrifically bad things happening to these people all at once. The universe seems to dole out all of the good at once and then all of the bad at once. It doesn't seem particularly well thought out.

Take Riley, for instance. She was a golden retriever cross with no eyes. She lost them both to glaucoma years ago. To avoid the freaky sunken orbit look after her eyes were removed, prostheses (which look like rubber balls) were placed in the empty eye sockets at the time of her surgery and the skin was closed over them. It just looked like she was choosing to walk around with her eyes closed, not like she'd had both eyes removed. A few years later, she developed a nasty tumour in one of her eye sockets (around one of her prosthetic eyeballs) and her owners brought her in for a consultation.

There was something special about Riley. She seemed to look right at you and responded to her environment like a sighted dog. When I was around her, I felt like I was in the presence of an old soul. We talked to Riley's owners about our recommendations. They agreed to do a CT scan of her head and chest, as well as a surgery—called an orbitectomy—to remove the tumour. The clients wanted us to do anything for Riley. They told me that she meant everything to them.

In fact, she was everything to them. She was all they had left. A few weeks prior, they'd had a house fire in the middle of the night and Riley, their blind dog, woke up the entire household by barking and running around. She saved her family from the fire. Everyone got out safely, but the house was destroyed. The owners told me, "We don't have a house any more, but we have our Riley." They'd already loved her immensely even before she became a hero. She could do amazing things for a blind dog, like rollerblading. Her owner would take her out on his blades and she would run ahead, pulling him and navigating her way along the paved trails. Riley could see things that I couldn't. I hoped she knew that I was trying to help her, and I sensed she did—she recognized me when I walked into the room and would wag her tail and look my way.

Riley had a very big surgery to remove the tumour, some of the bone of her orbit, and a lot of skin and soft tissue. She recovered in our ICU. Luckily, her owners were not worried about how she looked, and they had already grieved her lost vision long ago. They took her home after a few days in hospital. When her histopathology results came back, the surgical margins were clear of tumour, which was great news. Her cancer was unlikely to come back locally. However, the pathologist noted that the tumour had a very aggressive microscopic appearance, suggesting that there was a high risk of distant metastasis, or spread. We recommended chemotherapy for her, but the owners declined. They were financially tapped out and trying to pick up the pieces of their lives. It was heartbreaking.

I lost touch with these owners. They may have felt embarrassed because they couldn't afford to continue with all the recommended care for Riley now that the financial reality of the house fire and Riley's diagnosis had sunk in. I know that she did well for months, but I am not sure what happened after that. I hope she is still with her family, rollerblading and watching over them.

I also had a client who was blind. Like Riley, he'd had both of his eyes removed. His dog, Duchess, a pitbull, had a tumour in her lower eyelid that had been removed a few years prior and then recurred. The owner had lost so much in a short period of time: he told me his wife had recently left him and taken their children. His only remaining family member was his mother, who had just died. He'd only recently lost his vision. Duchess was all he had left. I talked to him on the phone a lot about his options for Duchess. He had many barriers to treatment—mostly financial—but also practical. It was hard for him to get his dog to us for appointments; hard for him to monitor her for complications associated with treatment; and hard for him to come back in quickly if problems developed. His options were to do nothing; do a moderate surgery followed by radiation treatment; or do a radical resection of the tumour, eye, and surrounding bone. He opted for the second option. He was not ready to let her go. This was a good option for him, but it meant Duchess would have to stay in hospital for a month and have radiation treatment after surgery.

It was around Christmas when we were talking over the phone about his options. He was alone and had nobody to help bring in Duchess for surgery until after the holidays. We planned her surgery for the new year and, signing off on the phone, I reflexively told him to have a good Christmas. Sometimes I am such an asshole. As soon as the chirpy words fell out of my mouth, I wished I could take them back. The thing is, I am not even that into Christmas. I don't find it all that magical. But I am pretty certain that a man with limited resources who has recently lost his vision and his entire family, and whose dog has recurrent cancer that he can barely afford to treat, is not going to have a holly-jolly Christmas this year. I heard him choke up on the other end of the line as he managed to get out the obligatory response—that he hoped I would have a merry Christmas, too. I teared up as I got off the phone. Duchess came in after Christmas, as planned, and had surgery followed by radiation. She was a calm, sweet dog and she handled her treatments well. Before long she was back home with her dad and cancer-free.

There seems to be an inverse correlation between the number of terrible things going on in people's lives and how polite they are when they come to their veterinarian. Some clients with lots of money and a sick pet (which is admittedly very stressful) will fall apart if things do not go exactly as planned or exactly as they want them to go. They can be demanding and difficult to please. Small delays or changes in the plan turn into massive problems, guilt trips, and misdirected anger at people who are bending over backwards trying to make things work behind the scenes. Technicians, front desk staff, and interns are easy prey to unload on. On the other hand, the people who are suffering multiple tragedies simultaneously, the ones whom I would excuse for these antics, are, as a whole, calm and polite. Maybe it's that they have perspective, or that nothing surprises them any more, or that they don't expect things to go well, so when they don't, there is no reaction.

I KNOW THIS IS a book about dogs, but here is one cat story. When I met Lily's mom, Astrid, she was anxious but polite, and very happy to be at our hospital. She interrupted me a lot—every time I tried to get through something she cut me off. So I backed off and let her talk. She had cancer, too. Her mother had died of metastatic colon cancer and that is when she got her kitten, Lily. On a routine evaluation for familial colon disease, Astrid was also diagnosed with metastatic colon cancer. She had surgery and was undergoing chemotherapy. Her ashen complexion and thinning hair made sense to me now, as well as her angst about Lily. Lily was a feisty 2.8-kilogram, ten-year-old cat who could not be examined when she was awake because she was so aggressive in the hospital. A lot of perfectly reasonable cats act like rabid wild animals when they are in the hospital. Lily was a handful. She had been seen the week before by our oncology service and had all of her tests done when she was under general anesthetic, including a CT scan of her chest.

Lily had a history of laboured breathing and had been diagnosed with a large mass in her chest called a thymoma. She needed surgery to remove it. It's a big surgery for a little cat, but there weren't a lot of other options. She needed to get better so she could help Astrid get through what she now referred to as the "darkest days of my life." The owner needed some time to think about what she wanted to do. We had a counsellor on staff and I went to find her to help Astrid with her decision-making.

I relayed the owner's background to our counsellor: the client's mother had died of colon cancer and now the client had metastatic colon cancer, and the cat also had cancer.

I started crying. The counsellor paused and asked me if I needed to sit down and talk. That's great, our counsellor thought I needed counselling. I told her I was fine but that the whole situation was just really sad.

I think I would need counselling if I didn't cry from time to time with this job. A counselling service is relatively new in veterinary medicine. The bottom line is that a lot of our clients need help to make decisions. If they don't have a trained counsellor to talk to, they will make use of the nearest veterinarian or technician, but we don't have the same skills and, unfortunately, we don't usually have the time.

Some clients are instantly offended when I suggest that they talk to our counsellor. They think that I think they are crazy, and that is why I am running for the nearest mental health professional. But they definitely need someone to talk to, someone to help them, just without the stigma attached. Sometimes we all need a paid friend to help us through difficult times. I always used to ask clients if they would like to talk to our counsellor, but now I just bring them in, introduce everyone, and then leave them to it. I know that trained social workers can smooth out whatever awkwardness I have created in my wake. No client has ever complained about having someone to talk to who cares about them. We want our clients to feel like they have made the best decision for themselves and their pets. I left Lily's mom and the counsellor to it for a few hours. It was hard for her. Her life was pretty complicated. In the end, she opted for surgery.

Lily's surgery went well. I was superstressed. I felt like I had more than just little Lily riding on this, like her mom's happiness and successful treatment outcome. Lily was a tough cat. Her feistiness made her hard to handle, but it also made her fight and recover quickly from surgery. When Astrid visited, we had to dress her up in a gown and gloves. We weren't protecting Lily, we were protecting her mom because she was immunosuppressed. There is so much more to think about when multiple family members have cancer.

It happens more often than you would think. More than one person in the household gets cancer and then the dog or cat gets cancer. My mother has reported to me that her dog park friends were discussing this phenomenon and apparently the latest dog park wisdom is that this is due to "sympathetic cancers." I need to dispel this myth right now. There is no such thing as "sympathetic cancer." Our pets are wonderful; they give us companionship and love, and they serve us in so many ways. They may even be able to detect cancer, but getting cancer just because we have cancer is not something that our pets do. There are a few legitimate reasons for this observation. There is a lot of cancer out there. We are all living longer (people and animals) because of advances in health care, and so we all live long enough to get cancer. We also live in the same environment as our pets, so we expose them to the same things that may cause our cancers. Beyond that, it is just bad luck. Lily and her mom recovered together at home over the summer. Her mom went back to work as a teacher and Lily went back to keeping her mom company and terrorizing veterinarians. Things can always get worse, but they can get better, too.

ACCOMPANYING THE UPLIFTING WISDOM that things could always be worse, there is an emerging school of thought that suggests I should just get comfortable with the idea of living with a cancer diagnosis. I should accept that cancer and I are moving in together. I didn't think it was such a good idea, but cancer insisted. My doctor also suggested it. He said that I would be "living with my cancer," and I have decided to hate this expression, even though I have used it myself in the past. Now people can "live *with* their cancer" and "die *with* their cancer," rather than "*of* their cancer," and everyone thinks that this is such a clever and refreshing way to look at cancer. When people say it, they put a lot of emphasis on *with*, so you know that this subtle and cunning switch of a tiny preposition is making a *world* of difference to *my* cancer experience. I'm confused. Am I supposed to befriend my cancer or join the war against it? Should we be peaceful or violent with cancer? I guess it depends on what kind of cancer you have. If you have good cancer, you should be peaceful because you are going to be fine and getting violent is not going to serve you. If you have bad cancer, you should be peaceful because you are going to die and getting violent is not going to serve you.

There is a new line of thinking in oncology. As long as they move slowly, grow slowly, and generally behave themselves, the cancer cells that have inhabited your otherwise healthy body get to stay. Everyone likes this plan, except possibly the people who are living and dying *with* these uninvited guests. It is not very helpful to be told that a cluster of thyroid cancer cells could hang out in my lymph nodes for months or even years and never cause a problem, and not to worry about it. Am I just supposed to know they are there and do nothing about it? No, thank you. I want them gone. They need to be cut out, nuked, or poisoned. They are not welcome here, and living with them is driving me crazy. Maybe it is just me. Maybe I am not a very inspiring cancer patient.

It makes much more sense to apply this happy logic to dogs and cats. All dogs and cats understand is their quality of life. They don't feel fear when they are diagnosed. They don't worry about death. They don't worry about chemotherapy or losing a leg. Most people think that dogs undergoing chemotherapy will become the classic emaciated cancer patients. The truth is, our canine chemo patients usually gain weight during their treatment, because their owners feed them anything they want. People also think that their pets will lose their hair, but because most pets have fur, not hair, most of them keep their coats. For those that don't, there are a lot of cute outfits they can wear, once their owners get over the shock of their dog looking like an alien.

Dogs and cats live for the moment and find joy in everyday things. We can learn from this. If you could slow cancer down to the point where it wouldn't affect a dog or cat's quality of life, many really could die *with* their cancer. That is, if they don't live for too long (which they don't, compared to humans) and if the cancer moves very slowly. Dogs also won't have to go through the irritation of someone telling them that they are going to live *with* their cancer, because they won't understand this sentence, which is a blessing. The grief and stress are still very present in veterinary oncology, but it is felt by the owners, so it is grief and stress once removed.

FOUR WEEKS AFTER THE "you have cancer" phone call from my surgeon, I am at my post-diagnosis appointment. My surgeon tells me about the next steps. First, I need surgery to remove the rest of the thyroid gland. We also talk about radioactive iodine treatment, which has its pros and cons. If we don't do the radioactive iodine and the cancer does come back or metastasize, my surgeon says we will just do more surgery and/or I will have to take radioactive iodine. He is pretty blasé about it, as though it is no big deal to come out of remission, get the diagnosis that you are out of remission, and then navigate your way through our health care system again to get your recurrent metastatic cancer treated. As if it was all so easy the first time around.

Mortality means you die from your disease. *Morbidity* is how much crap you have to deal with to keep it at bay. It's great to hear that I am unlikely to die from this cancer. I am lucky and I know it. This happy news helps me and those around me not take this all too seriously. I have cancer lite. However, I am still worried about the morbidity part. Cancer is becoming my full-time job and it already was my full-time job. Cancer takes up all of my time. I vote for more crap now and no crap later, rather than a slow trickle of crap to "live with" until I die *of* or *with* it.

My surgeon tells me that living *with* this cancer will be much like living *with* rheumatoid arthritis. I think back to the dogs with rheumatoid arthritis that I have treated; their joints were completely eroded, and I watched the crippling, progressive pain that they went through, and saw how they could barely walk. It was heartbreaking and hopeless. I also think about a few people I have known with this terrible disease. To be fair, there are new treatments, but it does not sound like an appealing comparison. Rheumatoid arthritis makes thyroid cancer look like a cakewalk. I start laughing and tell him that he might want to pick something else to be his poster disease for living with a chronic disease. Living *with* your thyroid cancer will be like living *with* AIDS. Maybe they even say that about AIDS now (living *with* it). Maybe leprosy? Drug-resistant TB? Crohn's disease? Sounds great, bring on the cancer.

I had other plans for my living arrangements with thyroid cancer. I was hoping for surgery, then a nice big dose of radiation. I want to break up with this cancer and never see it again. Maybe I gave cancer the wrong idea because of all the time that I have spent with it over the years. Sure, I have found cancer fascinating, exciting, and dramatic. We used to be very close and we now have a lot in common, but I want to kick it out of my body and never see it again. I think that the more aggressive the breakup, the more likely it will be to stay away. I am worried that if I don't do the radioactive iodine, it may be misinterpreted as an invitation to come back; tacit approval to inhabit the same space as me again, like a flirty text with an open invitation to get in touch or to stay friends. I have to tell cancer that no means no.

If I am going to live *with* my cancer, I want to know everything about it. Tell me everything, cancer. Start at the beginning and leave nothing out. I start reading the "Revised American Thyroid Association Management Guidelines for Patients with Thyroid Nodules and Differentiated Thyroid Cancer" in the journal *Thyroid* (yes, there is an entire medical journal called *Thyroid*). I am lucky that I can understand it. Most people with cancer flail around on the Internet and grapple to understand what is happening to their bodies. I cringe when I see some of the thyroid cancer blogs. The intentions are always good but the information is a bit misguided. I don't feel that physicians take the same amount of time to explain to their patients what is happening as I do for my clients.

Once you have a cancer diagnosis, cancer will be with you forever, like a ghost. It might be a friendly ghost, like Casper the friendly thyroid cancer, or a terrifying one that haunts you and frightens you to death, like the *Changeling* ghost, but it is always going to be there. You don't get to decide what kind of ghost it is—that is dependent on the disease and, to some extent, your treatment; where you live; if you have a good doctor; if they took action quickly; if it's treatable; if you advocated for yourself; and if you fought.

There is so much pressure to fight cancer. As if you could fight it off yourself. We are at war with cancer, and we are all fighting. There are more than a few problems with this concept. The word *cancer* is tarnished. We fear the word instinctively, the same way we fear spiders and snakes. We can try to fight cancer, win the war, end all childhood cancers, and end breast cancer. We can run, jump, bike, walk for the cure. We can even say "Fuck Cancer" and buy T-shirts and stickers with the same slogan, just because it makes us feel better and makes us feel tougher than the disease. But none of that will really solve anything, because we are not tougher than this disease. Fighting cancer is a bit like fighting world poverty or fighting war. (Let's start a war on war!) Cancer, poverty, and war are all vast problems that are diverse and complex. Cancer is hundreds of diseases that are given one name. We have given them an umbrella term but we do not have an umbrella cause or an umbrella solution. We have collectively decided that we don't like the concept of mortality and we would prefer not to die, but we all have to die at some point. The race to end all cancers is really a race for immortality.

All this fighting gets pretty tiring. You are already sick and going through treatment. You have to fight to get through our health care system and then you have to fight the cancer, too? I hear the war drums beating their anti-cancer rhetoric, but I'm way too tired. And what if

I lose? Did I not fight enough? Is that what people will think? Was I too negative? Did the negative thoughts kill me? What about the negative thoughts that I thought when I was fighting like a girl?

People like to think that if you have a more positive outlook you can beat your cancer. However, a recent study suggested that thinking positively has no effect on survival for cancer patients. No one wants to hear this—it's too depressing. We want to believe that if we think positively and face this disease bravely we can fight it, beat it, and cure it. Before the big scandal, we believed that Lance Armstrong beat the odds because he was a powerful athlete and because of his will to survive; or was it because he had a potentially curable disease and the best possible medical care? We expect famous people to be survivors because they are famous people. They are larger than life and they are all winners. There are actually famous people who don't survive cancer. They are just not available to make an appearance on the talk-show circuit to share the experience and their inspirational fight. If you are not a cancer winner, are you a cancer loser?

What about the people who have succumbed to cancer? What about my friend's fourteen-year-old son who loved biking and Lance Armstrong (again, pre-scandal). He had leukemia and I was sure he would survive. The prognosis is usually good. He bravely faced his multiple bouts of chemotherapy, fungal pneumonia, and ultimately his own death. His acceptance that his death was inevitable was heartbreaking. Was he just not positive enough? If he had just been more optimistic, could he have fought and won? I have three friends whose mothers died of cancer recently and a friend whose father has metastatic colon cancer. Not enough positivity?

What about Jack Layton—the plucky, brave, great left-wing politician whom I watched become leader of the opposition as I recovered from my first surgery in a historic Canadian election? He was dead within months of the unprecedented results, struck down at the peak of his career by a second, aggressive form of head and neck cancer. Canadians across the country mourned the loss of a politician who had just started to initiate real change. Did all of these people just not try hard enough? Did they not have enough hope or courage? This is the danger of thinking that our attitude can chart the course of a disease. It can leave already devastated families even more devastated because they will feel that their loved one may have lacked the will to survive.

How we face cancer as patients and families is really just a reflection of how we face the ups and downs of life. Obviously cancer is a major down, but our attitude toward diagnosis and treatment will make a major difference to our quality of life. This is where the positivity will come in. Positivity may not be able to change the outcome, but it can change the experience. As a family member or friend to someone with cancer, our attitude will also have a major impact on the patient's enjoyment of life. For my veterinary patients, this is easier because quality of life is everything. Living for the moment is everything. For me, quality of life is everything, too. For human cancer patients, this diagnosis usually makes us pause, at least for a little while, and try to assess if we are happy, and ask ourselves what is really important.

Maybe we need to redefine what it means to win or lose with cancer. All cancers are not created equal. Even within one type of cancer, sometimes it is treatable and sometimes it is not, despite the best efforts of doctors, patients, and families. Sometimes life and cancer deal you a bad hand. How you play your cards may be more important than anything else.

VETERINARY MEDICINE HAS SO many options for personalized treatment, but one of the most common questions I get asked is "What would you do if it was your dog?" The options for my patients range from euthanasia to palliative treatments to full-on curative-intent therapies. Many of our clients are terrified of making mistakes and they are often too emotional to make good decisions. Complicating things further, most clients feel that they are being judged. This is because they are being judged. By everyone. There is a wide range of opinions on how to treat animals with cancer. This would be fine if everyone would be just a little bit shyer about asking personal questions and offering up their uninformed two cents about the choices my clients make for their pets and the expense involved. It's not really worth trying to explain to a non-animal person what your dog means to you. You can't. It's kind of like how new parents tell childless people that they can never understand the parent–child bond, and how the love they share with their new baby is the greatest, purest love in the world. I think that, on some level, they do this in order to make barren couples (like the one I'm part of) aware that they will never experience a love like that and, basically, feel as though our lives have no purpose. At least I remain blissfully ignorant of how great my life could be, and I really dig my dog.

I do my best to dodge the question of what I would do if it were my dog. It is not my dog, so I can't really answer. I try to help my clients by getting them to focus on their goals and limitations. This will usually lead to a good plan. Sometimes the goals are not reasonable. For example, I had a client with an eighteen-year-old cat in renal failure, with lung cancer, who told me that he would like to go ahead with treatment and was hoping his cat would live for another five or six years. Your treatment goal cannot be a miracle, but it can be long-term control, a good quality of life and, sometimes, even a cure. Cancer treatment means redefining success.

The limitations can be financial, but it's not always about money. Sometimes the limitations are time-related, or related to the other things that are going on in a client's life. I recently saw a golden retriever with a large sarcoma on his head. It probably could have been removed and the dog cured, if we had seen them sooner, but they let it get so big that even a radical surgery was unlikely to have a good long-term outcome. Usually this type of delay stems from neglect, a lack of funds, or ignorance and fear. But in this golden retriever's case, it was none of those things. The owners had an eight-year-old son with leukemia who was undergoing chemotherapy, and they just couldn't juggle everything. They were exhausted, and now, on top of everything, they felt guilty about their dog, whom they all loved dearly, especially their son. They knew that delaying therapy for their dog was going to mean a worse prognosis for him. All I could do was move forward and say, "Well, he is here now."

I saw my most extreme case of a mass gone awry when I was a senior veterinary student. I helped take care of an exceptionally aggressive husky with a humungous tumour that extended from his shoulder down his upper leg. The mass was bigger than his head. It wasn't really bothering him until it got large enough that it outgrew its own blood supply and the tumour tissue began to die. The necrotic tumour opened up and stinky fluid started to drip out of it. The dog could turn his head to chew on this "second head," and he managed to rupture one of the large blood vessels supplying the tumour. The owners found him in his run, lying in a pool of his own blood. He almost bled to death and showed up at our teaching hospital in emergency. He was in shock due to the severe blood loss. He was treated with several blood transfusions and we removed the tumour and amputated his leg. The tumour was so big that this was the only option for treatment. The expense and what this dog went through were all exponentially greater than what would have been necessary if the owners had treated the mass when it was small. They could have had a four-legged dog and likely a cure for a fraction of the cost, and much less of an ordeal for all concerned. The owners, however, appeared thrilled with the outcome and offered no explanation for letting the mass get so large.

Sometimes it is hard to tell why a client holds off on treatment until late in the course of the disease. It happens in human patients, too. They let things go. They watch a large tumour grow in their abdomen and figure that they are getting a bit fat, even though their abdomen is hard as a rock. Denial is a powerful force, but you have to think they must know that, whatever it is growing on them-selves/their dog, it is not good and it needs attention.

THE SECOND MOST COMMON question that owners ask me when they are trying to decide on treatment options is "Am I putting him through too much?" Nobody who loves their dog would want to put him through too much. The problem is that we have no way of defining what "too much" means and who gets to decide. Even within our own profession, this debate rages on. A recent bout of letters to the editor in the *Canadian Veterinary Journal* contained a nasty volley of insults from two general practitioners toward all veterinary oncologists, accusing the whole specialty of playing God with no thought to the welfare of our patients, recommending extreme treatments that are painful and unpleasant, with little benefit. Their comments were hurtful, polarizing, and irresponsible. A debate that starts out in this vein has all the trappings of American politics: nobody wins and our patients always lose. How can our clients decide what is best for their pets when veterinarians can't come to a consensus on what is an appropriate level of care for cancer treatment in animals and what constitutes "too much"? The answer is a moving target made up of the individual medical details of the case, finances, the owner's beliefs, the veterinarian's beliefs, facilities available, and, somewhere in there, the patient's personality—we do our best to do what we think they would want.

Clients may perceive that a procedure or treatment is too much to put their dog through, without realizing that doing nothing could be far worse. The most classic example of this in veterinary surgical oncology is osteosarcoma, or bone cancer, of the limb. The most common treatment recommendation for osteosarcoma in dogs is amputation of the limb, and most dogs will handle this very well. I have amputated hundreds of dogs' legs for bone cancer. The surgery takes less than an hour and the vast majority of these dogs are more comfortable immediately after surgery than they were in the weeks leading up to surgical treatment. How can that be? Bone cancer pain is very difficult to treat with the medications available for people and animals. Post-operative pain, on the other hand, is relatively easy to treat. I feel like this is communicated to me by almost every patient that is relieved of their bone cancer pain with an amputation. After surgery, the dog's grimace is gone, replaced by bright eyes and a dog's smile. I feel like they would sit up and say thank you if they could. That is not to say that they are normal, because having three legs is not normal, but having cancer is not normal either. Humans and dogs with cancer, and their people, have to find a new normal.

The applicable yet overused vet cliché in this illustration is that dogs come with "three legs and a spare." I feel sorry for people who still laugh when they hear this or repeat it thinking it is a new one, not realizing how many times this lame vet joke has been told. A real knee-slapper. There is truth to it, though. Most dogs will thrive on three legs. But no matter how much education you give, or how many videos of three-legged dogs you show on YouTube, some clients cannot accept a three-legged dog. Even if the leg is fractured, painful, and useless to the dog, clients are more attached to the body part than their dog.

Clients don't just get attached to limbs. (Here comes the obligatory veterinary testicle stories of the book.) Testicles are another body part that some clients have difficulty letting go of, and usually those clients are men. They get attached to their dogs and then to their dog's testicles. They equate neutering their dog to neutering themselves. They could never do that to their best friend (i.e., their own balls). The first neuter I performed as a senior veterinary student was a covert operation. The owner brought her three-year-old bichon frisé to our veterinary teaching hospital to have him neutered while her husband was out of town. Her husband was adamantly opposed to his not-at-all manly dog being further emasculated. The neuter went fine but I didn't close the tunica, which is the sac that surrounds the testicles. In young dogs, this is not a problem. In an adult dog, like this one, the tunica can have well-developed blood vessels. I learned the valuable lesson that it is better to close the tunica in mature dogs to prevent bleeding. This dog developed enough bleeding that his scrotum (the skin that previously housed his testicles) filled with blood and became twice its normal size and dark purple. It was a huge, dark, purple sac hanging between the hind legs of a small, white, fluffy dog. The clandestine part of the mission had failed.

It's not just men who get attached to their dog's testicles. One of my classmates in veterinary school had a client tell her that she wouldn't neuter her dog because she liked to play with his testicles when they sat on the couch and watched TV together. This is definitely too much information. People, love your pets, but don't *love* your pets. Something about the white coat, stethoscope, and clinical setting of a veterinary clinic makes people talk. Most clients feel very comfortable with their veterinarian, which is good, but sometimes they get a little too comfortable and they start to feel free to discuss their own bodies and/or medical conditions, which is very, very bad. We are veterinarians for a reason. Suddenly, personal details about their health and/or body parts are flowing out of them and there is no way to stop it. I had a client once tell me that her dog's ear infection smelled similar to when she got an infection "down there" (gesturing toward her crotch/vagina). Wow. That is very helpful. I think I need to excuse myself.

We are also sometimes in the awkward position of removing personal items from dogs' stomachs. These are the stories that we like to tell each other at vet parties: the mortifying tampon, women's underwear, women's underwear that did not belong to the "lady" of the house (awkward), and a cock ring removed from the stomach of a police dog after a raid on a "massage parlour."

My favourite intimate client story is not one of my own. It did not take place in a sterile small animal clinic but in a dairy barn, with a colleague of my husband's who is a large animal veterinarian. The farmer had recently had a vasectomy. Just as the veterinarian was turning away from his bovine patient (yes, after putting his arm up her bum), his client dropped trou in the middle of the barn to ask if his junk looked okay. His testicles were swollen, purple, and the size of grapefruits. They were so large that they obscured all but the very tip of his penis. Do you really need a medical professional to tell you that this is not okay? In the spirit of one medicine, here is a good principle that translates to all species: if you have lost sight of your genitals for any reason, you need to seek immediate medical attention.

But enough about testicles. Most of us agree that they are optional items, at least in dogs. Despite what people might think, there is actually a long list of organs and body parts that are superfluous to veterinary (and, I imagine, human) surgical oncologists: one or two legs (as mentioned), one or two eyes, one or two ears, a lung, large amounts of liver, a kidney, up to seven ribs, the bladder, the prostate, the penis, two-thirds of the tongue, the spleen, the mandible and large portions of the skull, to name a few. There is a lot of redundancy built into the system. I worked with a veterinary surgeon who removed his own dog's spleen, tonsils, uterus, ovaries, and anal sacs when she was a puppy, just to have a few less items kicking around in which to develop cancer. It's extreme cancer prevention.

When I was a surgery resident, we had a team of TV reporters from *W5*, the Canadian investigative journalism show, visit our teaching hosptial. Most of the clinicians I worked with refused to talk to them or be on camera. They were convinced that the *W5* team was only there to do recon for an hour-long special highlighting the

exorbitant cost of veterinary care and portraying veterinarians in the worst possible light (which actually does happen all the time and is often misguided or mean-spirited.)
At the time, I was more trusting; I was open and willing
to talk. Frankly, I am a media whore and I wanted to be
on TV. The crew followed me through the drama of a dog
that was hit and dragged by a car. The dog had a large
wound on his abdomen that also encompassed his penis,
which was mangled beyond repair and needed to go. So I
amputated a dog's penis on national television; it is now
my claim to fame. My mother-in-law still shows this video
to her friends any chance she gets. It is real-life vet hospital
drama. After the surgery, the earnest television reporter
interviewed me beside my recovering penis-less patient.
She asked me, in all seriousness, "So, is he a girl now?"
This is near the top of my all-time stupidest questions list.
I said something like, "No, he is still a boy," but I wanted
to respond, "If I remove your tits, are you now a man?"

I have had a few body parts removed myself. When I
was seventeen, I had my tonsils out. At twenty-seven, I had
my gallbladder removed. Now, at thirty-eight, I am having my entire thyroid gland out. Every decade or so I shed
some extraneous glandular tissue that has been causing
me grief. I am not sure what will be next. Maybe it will be
my boobs. Angelina Jolie just lost her breasts in a courageous and very public prophylactic double mastectomy. Her
risk of developing breast cancer was considered extremely
high, so why not have them removed and replaced with
a new, perfect pair? Breasts that are new, perky, cancer-
free, and free from the toll of gravity and breastfeeding the
Jolie-Pitt soccer team. This sounds like a good plan to me.

Removing a dog's jaw for cancer is common, but it can be a difficult decision to get your head around if it is your dog. Jake was a nine-and-a-half-year-old male mixed breed who developed a fast-growing sarcoma on his lower jaw. His owners were Joan and Susan, two raucous women who had just retired. Like any old married couple, they bickered, chatted, and laughed during Jake's consultation. Joan talked a lot and asked so many questions, and Susan told her to stop talking and asking the very busy doctor so many questions. Their love for each other and Jake was obvious. They told me that Jake was their companion, their security, a way for them to meet new people, and that he kept them healthy because he forced them to go on walks every day. When their previous dog died of kidney disease, they had decided not to get another dog because it hurts too much when they die. But they found themselves at the Humane Society two months later, "just looking around," and that is when they found Jake in a litter of ten.

They were on a fixed income and Jake's disease hit them hard financially. That part was harder for them to manage than losing Jake's jaw, but they didn't want to lose him and they found a way to go ahead. Jake had some preliminary tests and a CT scan. He then had a mandibulectomy, during which most of his lower jaw was removed. We took the tumour and a wide margin of surrounding bone to make sure we got it all. Jake stayed in the hospital for two nights after surgery. It took him only thirty-six hours to start eating canned food. Most dogs are very motivated to eat and they will not let something like missing a large portion their jaw prevent them from chowing down. The owners felt that he was his normal happy self following the surgery, and after three weeks they reported that he was swimming and fetching his Frisbee again. (The owners were instructed that he not be allowed to play with toys for a month, but what can you do?) They fed Jake by wetting down his kibble and placing it on a rubber mat to give him some traction. He would turn his head and scoop up the food with his tongue and the few lower teeth that remained.

When Jake's jaw was assessed by the pathologist, the margins of excision were clean, which suggested that recurrence of tumour in his mouth was unlikely. However, the tumour was considered a high-grade sarcoma, which meant there was a 40 to 50 percent chance of metastasis to another site in the future. In this situation, chemotherapy is recommended. The owners declined. Surgery was the one shot they wanted to give Jake, and that decision had been hard enough. The finances and philosophy of chemotherapy just didn't fit for them.

Six months after Jake's treatment, I got an email update from his moms:

Subject: hi Dr. Sarah

Hi Dr. Sarah!

I hope things are going well for you.

I just wanted you to know that Jake has developed more growths in his mouth. I have attached some photos for you. Just like the other tumours, they grew really fast. I

know there is nothing to be done now, but do you think
we should contact the hospital, so that they can update
his file?

Happy trails,
Joanie

I was surprised and sad to read this news and, as the
surgeon who had attempted to cure him with a radical
surgery, it was hard not to feel terrible and wonder if I
should have taken more tissue or done something differ-
ently. Luckily, the owners attached several pictures of
Jake and his growths. The masses didn't look like tumour
regrowth to me. It looked more like an accumulation of
saliva under his jaw. This is a potential complication after
a mandibulectomy.

I wrote back:

Subject: re: hi Dr. Sarah

Dear Joan,

Thank you for the update and the pictures.

I think it would be a very good idea for you to get in
touch with the oncology department.

Has a veterinarian looked at Jake? This may be growth
recurrence, but it is also possible that he has a condition
called a sialocele, which is an accumulation of saliva
that can occur with blocked salivary ducts. I don't want

to create false hope, since I have not seen Jake, but I would strongly recommend that either your veterinarian or one of our oncologists take a look at this to figure this out. A sialocele would feel quite soft and a recurrence of tumour would feel firm.

Please keep me updated.

Sincerely,
Sarah Boston

Luckily, they listened to this advice. (*Spoiler alert: in the time between Jake's surgery and his recheck, I had moved from my position in Ontario to a position at the University of Florida.*) I wasn't able to see Jake myself for his recheck, but he did go back to the oncology department.

Subject: re:re: hi Dr. Sarah

Hi Dr. Sarah,

Jake went in this morning. You were right, Jake has blocked salivary glands—no cancer. Jake goes into surgery tomorrow morning to help saliva drainage. Hopefully all goes well.

Thank you so much for your support and advice.

Happy trails,
Joanie

Jake had a simple surgery to drain this fluid accumulation and was back to himself within a day. I was thankful that the owners had updated me. I can't imagine what they were thinking and going through watching those "growths" come back. That is not to say that it can't happen. A report of clean margins from the pathologist makes a surgical oncologist feel brilliant, but the reality is that they cannot possibly evaluate every millimetre of the surgical margin, so even when the margin is called clean, recurrence is a possibility. I got an update from Joan and Susan a few months later. There were more pictures. This time Jake was at the lake, carrying a massive stick in his mouth and looking quite proud—quite a feat if most of your lower jaw is missing. He'd wrapped his tongue around the bottom of the stick, like a giraffe, to keep it in place. Jake was not about to let his cancer stand in the way of something as important as carrying his stick around at the lake. His owners sent me an email on the one-year anniversary of his surgery to tell me that he was still his "happy-go-lucky self" and thanking me for everything. Two weeks later, I received another email:

Subject: sad news

Dear Dr. Sarah,

Yesterday, Jake suffered a tragic accident at the horse farm.

I had hired a rodeo rider to come to the horse farm to ride my high-strung horse. When a large farm tractor

came by, my horse went into a bucking frenzy by the
gate where Jake was resting. It happened so fast that I
don't know if it was the rider or the horse that crushed
his hind end, but the end result is that Jake's left hip
was dislocated and his right ankle was shattered. He was
unable to get up or walk. I took Jake to the veterinary
hospital. With both hind legs damaged, the after-surgery
care would have been too much for him and us to deal
with. Jake's happy "signature Jake" bounce would be
gone forever.

We decided to have him euthanized this morning. Our
hearts are broken, and we are in shock. Just two weeks
ago, we were celebrating his one-year anniversary, after
surviving his jaw surgery. Words cannot express how
much we will miss him.

Please say a prayer for Jake and for us. May the angels
give us strength.

Joan

For the first time, she did not sign her email "Happy trails."

In the end, it was the trauma of his accident that was
too much for Jake and his moms, not his cancer or losing
his lower jaw. It was tragic for his family, with the silver
lining that he lived for a year cancer-free.

What would I do if it were my dog? I will never give
you a straight answer because there isn't one. The best I
can do is answer this question with more questions. What
will cause more regret: not trying, or trying with the risk

of a catastrophic failure? What is the goal? Cure or pal-
liation? Aggressive or passive? Swinging for the fence or
going quietly? Can you afford this? Do you have the time?
All of these questions will lead to an answer, but it will be
a different answer for everyone.

I HAVE TRADED IN my surgery greens and mojo again for a hospital gown and anxiety. I am recovering from my completion thyroidectomy. It took three months to get from the diagnosis of thyroid carcinoma to this surgery date. The second surgical procedure was much like the first. The first time I had my right thyroid and accompanying mass removed. This time, my entire left thyroid was removed to decrease the risk of cancer recurrence. I am still in Toronto, but I am at a different hospital this time.

My hospital roommate is a Polish woman who has just had reconstructive surgery after a mastectomy for breast cancer. She leaves for a while to have a shower, and there is a flurry of activity when she gets back. From what I can gather from the growing crowd around her on the other side of the curtain, which consists of three nurses and her husband, she has seen something that she doesn't like during her shower. She sounds scared.

One of the nurses has a look at her breast flap, an integral part of the reconstructive surgery and what seems to be the root of the problem. She says that she thinks it is normal, just bruised, but she will see if she can get the on-call doctor to come by and take a look. Then she leaves. The conversation should have ended there, but the other two nurses stay in the room and continue to look at the woman's purple breast-flap and talk to her about it in a way that clearly indicates she should stop worrying (i.e., complaining). This does not instill any confidence in my Polish roommate, because they also make it fairly obvious that they don't actually know if it is okay or not. The more they talk, the worse it gets. They manage to get her whipped up into a genuine frenzy.

The on-call plastic surgery resident shows up about thirty minutes into the inane breast-flap discussion. He is not happy to have been called in for something so trivial and he lets it be known. He takes a look at the flap and tells her it is normal bruising and should be okay. She doesn't speak perfect English, so to ensure that she understands what he is saying, he yells everything at her SLOWLY AND LOUD-LY, which upsets her further. He tells her it should be fine and that even if it isn't fine, they can't do anything about it right now anyway. He reminds her that he is supposed to be on call for true emergencies, not to be here talking to her about her non-urgent purple flap. This makes her feel bad, which is exactly what he intended. He tells her not to feel bad while she is crying and apologizing for bothering the very important doctor. It is like a case study of how not to communicate with a patient; how to make the patient feel like a pain in the ass; how to create a crisis out of nothing; and how to take a valid patient concern and escalate it into forty-five minutes of hysteria.

The surgery resident and accompanying entourage shuffle out of the room, leaving the patient weeping quietly and appropriately to herself. Her husband follows quickly behind the resident and I hear him in the hallway, apologizing to the doctor again for his wife's behaviour. Whose side is he on, anyway? Once things settle down, my roommate comes over to say hello to me and we get to talking like a couple of jailbirds about why we are here. She apologizes for the commotion. She is about my age. In the past two years, she has had every conceivable treatment for breast cancer.

It turns out she found a mass in her breast just after she arrived in Canada. It was 2 centimetres at the time and her GP did not get on it. She waited patiently. It took four and a half months for her to see a surgeon and get a diagnosis. She had no idea what to expect of our system, no understanding of her disease and the risks of waiting, and no one to help her. Despite the fact that her mass went from 2 centimetres to 11 centimetres and had metastasized to nine lymph nodes by the time she had her first surgery, she is still grateful to Canada for offering her treatment. She said that if she was still in Poland she would be dead by now, and did that cross thing across her chest for the Father, the Son, and the Holy Ghost. I guess it is a matter of perspective, but I don't think she has a lot to be happy about.

The Canadian health care system can take a serious health concern and drag things out for long enough that it becomes a life-threatening disease. Then, because the

system seems to function best when it is preventing imminent death, it swoops in and offers the most aggressive care
possible. And it's all free! My roommate has previously had
a full mastectomy and node dissection, radiation therapy,
and chemotherapy, and she's just had a breast reconstruction with a flap. She still would have needed treatment for
a 2-centimetre cancerous breast mass, but it would have
been so much less aggressive and so much easier on her.
The doses of surgery, chemo, and radiation she received
were all high, which comes at great physical and emotional
expense to the patient, not to mention putting a financial
burden on our health care system. Despite the aggressive
treatment, I suspect that her long-term prognosis is poor
and that she will die of this cancer, which might not have
been the case if she had been treated sooner. I tell her she
should consider a formal complaint against her GP. She
says that a lot of people have told her that, but I suspect
she doesn't have it in her. She is too tired.

I like my roomie a lot. She is good company. I pull out
my iPad and show her some of the pictures I have of axial
pattern flaps in dogs. This is similar to the type of flap that
she had for breast reconstruction. I show her pictures of
one of my patients that had a complication after a skin flap
was used to reconstruct a defect on his face, so that she
can see what a flap looks like when it is dead (black, cold,
and hard, not purple and warm like hers). I explain to her
that these kinds of flaps can get congested with blood as
they heal and this can make them purple, but that it should
resolve over the next few days. Her English is not as bad
as everyone thinks. She understands, and she seems a lot
more relaxed as she heads back to bed.

As for me, I haven't slept for a few days. I've had a bad morphine trip. There is a huge gash in my neck. I'm nauseous. My serum calcium has dropped below normal range. I'm twitching. I'm trying to quit the narcotics, and I've cried uncontrollably three times. It's been rough. This was surgery number two. It was supposed to be easier this time around. The tumour was already gone. I knew what to expect, and the hospital I'm in is bigger this time and has an international reputation for excellent care. This should have been no problem.

But let me go back to the beginning. My pre-surgical appointment started out very well. The pre-admission clinic ran like a well-oiled machine. I spent two and a half hours in a room and was visited by multiple nurses, a pharmacist, a lab tech, and an anesthesia resident. Everyone was polite, professional, knew their job, and knew about me. I was weighed, evaluated, measured, poked, auscultated, palpated, and swabbed. One of the nurses was able to maintain her decorum and never stopped making idle conversation with me and my husband while she inserted a swab into my rectum to test me for a hospital superbug called vancomycin-resistant enterococcus. Now that is professionalism.

Poppy, the primary pre-admission nurse in charge of the appointment, was lovely. She asked so many questions. I told her about the medication protocol for pain and nausea that I was on post-operatively for the first surgery and how it worked perfectly. I also mentioned that I didn't want to go home with codeine and that I was scared of being nauseous. Everything was recorded. Poppy even asked if there was anything that they could do to make my stay more comfortable. Wow! I felt as though I was going to be staying in a five-star hotel. I did the whole "I am always cold" routine I'd done many times already, and she assured me that they pile warm blankets on their patients post-operatively. She checked my surgery date and told me that she thought she would be there on my surgery day and would personally take good care of me. I was looking forward to it. I imagined Poppy wrapping pre-warmed blankets around me and taking the best care of me that she could. She made it sound as if there were a competition between the nurses to see whose patient was the warmest, happiest, most comfortable, and least nauseous post-op. Even the complimentary WiFi password at the hospital instilled confidence: "OurHealthCareIs#1."

The pre-admission appointment with Malice for my first surgery was frightening, and it made me apprehensive about the surgery. But as it turned out, my stay in the hospital and the care I received were incredible the first time around. The pre-admission appointment for my second surgery went perfectly, so I guess I should have known that this would have the opposite effect.

It started with a phone call from my surgeon at 7:24 a.m. It was all very disorienting. I was staying at a hotel two blocks from the hospital and I had planned a leisurely sleep-in and a stress-free stroll over to the hospital. My scheduled admission time was 11 a.m., with a surgery time of 1 p.m. That morning, the first patient on the surgery list for the day, who had likely waited months for his surgery date, decided to have breakfast. I'm sure he was told not to eat, but I guess he didn't understand or didn't remember. He was likely overloaded with information and stressed about his cancer diagnosis. Most people retain and understand only about 10 percent of what their doctor tells them, and the critical instruction to fast pre-operatively is not discussed in great detail. Maybe if they had told him he could die if he didn't fast for twelve hours before surgery, because the food in his stomach could find its way into his lungs when he was under anesthetic, the instructions would have stuck a little better.

With Mr. Breakfast wiped from the schedule for today, my surgeon called to see if I could come in early. I told him that I would rush in. As I hung up, I realized that I'd had a small glass of apple juice ten minutes before. I was allowed. I could have food up to midnight the night before and clear fluids up to five hours before my surgery. I was slightly obsessed with the fear that I would wake up hungry and/or dehydrated and/or nauseous after my surgery, so I had even set my alarm so I could wake up and drink my apple juice well before the five-hour clear fluid cut-off time and go back to sleep. I called the hospital back but had no way to get through to my surgeon. I told the receptionist about the apple juice situation, but he didn't know what to do. Terrified that I would lose my spot like Mr. Breakfast, I told him that I was on my way in and we could talk about it when I got there.

I rushed over, checked in, got changed, and then had to discuss my apple juice ingestion with several different nurses.

"How much?" they asked.

"About 200 millilitres."

"What time?"

"At 7:15 a.m."

I tried to explain that it really wasn't my fault, because I wasn't supposed to have surgery until 1 p.m. and I was trying to do them all a favour by showing up early, as the surgeon had requested, to make their day flow better. They seemed unimpressed with this excuse and annoyed by my juice indiscretion. There was judgement. I was nearly as stupid as the guy who ate breakfast, a selfish apple juice drinker who had screwed up their schedule for the second time in as many hours. I cringed as they relayed my apple juice stats around the pre-operative care unit. Then, just to be sure that everyone would know what I had done, one of the nurses took it upon herself to write this critical information on the whiteboard beside my name: Apple juice 200 mL — 7:15 a.m. I was mortified.

One of the anesthesiologists came by to see me and discuss the plan for the day, in light of apple-juice-gate. She was smiling and told me that she understood it wasn't my fault. I asked her if she would consider writing that on my forehead with permanent marker. Now I'm at the hospital three hours earlier than I need to be, my relaxing morning in the hotel room with my husband is gone, and I have to wait for a 1 p.m. table time anyway. I have annoyed everybody in the unit and I have nothing to do but sit there and watch the nurses and patients come and go in the pre-operative unit, all because of apple juice.

When things start happening, they happen fast. Once all traces of apple juice, and its accompanying shame, have left my stomach and the ward, a catheter is placed in my arm. Anesthesiologists are talking to me. My surgeon comes by for three seconds to talk. A dude with a do-rag starts wheeling me down to the OR. He tells me that he is fourteen hours into a twenty-hour shift. I am amazed that anyone can legally work a twenty-hour shift in a human hospital. He shrugs and tells me that he has to pay the mortgage somehow. My anesthesia is smooth and I'm out again.

Darkness for an undetermined period.

I'm back. I can feel the endotracheal tube in my trachea and I'm swallowing against it. Hello! Time to take the tube out! I can't say that due to said tube, but hope they notice me moving around. The anesthesiologist sees me chomping and swallowing on the tube and I can feel myself being extubated. It is a strange sensation and I think of all the dogs and cats who have felt this at my hands (we usually wait until they are almost chewing on the tube to be sure they can swallow and it is safe to extubate). The recovery nurse is pretty and cool. She is from Calgary and so am I. Somehow we are chatting about this connection. I tell her I am a vet and she asks me about turtles. I tell her what I know about turtle surgery, which isn't much. She is clearly fascinated by the parallels between turtle and human medicine. She is a good nurse and decides it is time to settle me in the ward. We pick up my husband en route and make our way to my room.

My ward nurse, Samara, is there. I tell her I am in pain. She is not around too much and I wait for just over an hour for pain medication. I know this because I am facing a clock and I have nothing else to do but stare at it. I get morphine, not the hydromorphone I had last time and specifically requested. They are similar drugs, but morphine has more potential side effects. Despite the fact that I told every health care worker I came into contact with *ad nauseum* pre-op—including the pre-admission nurse, the anesthesiologist, and my surgeon—that I wanted the same pain and anti-nausea medications for this surgery that I had for my first surgery, it does not happen. Interesting fact: they don't use hydromorphone as a first-line painkiller at this hospital, which nobody told me before my surgery. Even in my state, I know that this is a financial decision. Morphine is cheap, which is why they use it instead of its more expensive and proportionally more effective, and better-tolerated, counterpart hydromorphone.

I tell Samara that I had the same surgery three months ago and that I would like to ice my incision because it really helped last time. Maybe it's the morphine making me delusional, but I swear she rolled her eyes at me like a surly teenaged girl. She said, "Yeah, we don't do that here." I am trying to be nice, but I am not actually asking her opinion about the pros and cons of icing surgical sites post-operatively. I feel pretty capable of deciding that for myself. I just need some ice. Which came first, the angry patient on morphine or the nurse with a bad attitude? I still can't tell, but Samara and I have some bad chemistry and we are off to a poor start. The lovely Poppy told me that they would do whatever they could to make me more comfortable during my stay here. Why is it not playing out like that?

Samara reluctantly brings in the smallest bag of ice possible and tells me to be careful not to "burn" myself with it. That is ridiculous. I notice that she is wearing some sort of macramé cotton friendship bracelet. It is gross because (1) it is ugly and (2) (more important) there is no way to clean it or remove it. It is a perfect vehicle to transfer multiresistant superbugs from patient to patient. I can't take my eyes off it. Surgeons never stop thinking about germs. It is a blessing and a curse.

I'm on my own now. Superbug Samara is nowhere to be seen. I am trying to orient myself through the morphine and I'm noticing that morphine is not as good at controlling pain as hydromorphone, which is what I suspected. I am still in pain, feeling a bit nauseous, and in a really foul mood. I can hear an insanely loud program blasting from the next room over. Seriously? My husband gets up to see if he can do anything about the noise and comes back shaking his head. The noise is coming from the tablet of a patient who has just had pretty major surgery on his face and has no legs. Can't really ask him to turn it down, can you? He's also blind and, judging from the required volume of his in-room entertainment, almost deaf, too. It's a trap. I consider giving him my headphones, but then I will never want them back because of germs. I do feel bad for the guy—it sounds like he has pulled a very short straw—and I can appreciate that whatever he is listening to might well be his lifeline, but it is disturbing my not-peaceful recovery.

My nurse is gone and does not return until it is time to get me up to pee in the shared bathroom of my semi-private room. I am not sure what has been going on in here or who has been using this toilet, but the toilet seat is in no way clean and I am not talking about pee. I tell Samara that I can't/don't want to sit on a dirty toilet seat and ask if she can take me somewhere else. She tells me there are no other bathrooms that I can use. I find this hard to believe. She says that I have to pee right now but does not explain why it is such an emergency. Samara says that I can either squat over the toilet seat, using my quad strength alone (while on morphine and intravenous fluids, two hours after having a thyroidectomy); put some paper towel down and sit on it (which will surely result in strike-through of the fecal splatter and definite skin-to-poo contact — I am way too OCD for that, or maybe it is just normal to be repulsed by this idea); or pee into something called a hat (which looks remarkably like a hat, and is sitting on the germ-covered floor in the corner of the bathroom). I consider the hat option briefly, but I am certain that if I have to stand there holding the hat under myself, trying to pee into it while Samara monitors and records the event, it is not going happen for us. My urethral sphincter would never allow it. I can't even pee into my wetsuit when I'm scuba diving. I am aghast. The only option that I am considering is going back to bed and waiting until someone cleans the poo off the toilet seat.

Part of my surgical training involved developing the ability not to urinate for sixteen hours or more. I am confident that I could go back to bed and sleep for four hours and drink three cups of tea and a bottle of water, and then, maybe, I would need to pee. This is in the face of being on intravenous fluids. Speaking of which, it is curious to me that my intravenous fluids are not being regulated by a pump—a little machine that will allow you to set the rate of fluid administration per hour to the patient, and makes sure that the intravenous line does not block. Without a pump, you count the drip rate, do a bit of higher math, and hope for the best. Like hydromorphone, fluid pumps are expensive. Housekeeping staff to clean the toilets are also expensive in this first-world hospital that is being run like a third-world hospital. Socialized medicine at its finest.

It's not looking good for me. Samara is blocking the doorway, and the prospect of me going back to bed until she can solve my toilet-seat dilemma. I feel like I am being mugged for pee. I grab some paper towel and start cleaning the soiled toilet seat myself with soap and water. Apparently cleaning the toilet seat for me was not an option that she had considered. She left. I peed. I came out and asked her if she could get more paper towel for the bathroom (there was none left) and someone to clean the toilet. This did not happen during the remaining two days that I was in hospital. Although infection control and superbugs are a hot topic in the media, the solutions to these problems are often very simple: clean hands and toilets; no stinky cotton friendship bracelets or bacteria-harbouring, hideous false nails; plenty of paper towel to dry your hands after you wash them; and nurses who care and practice good hygiene are a start. Florence Nightingale had this figured out about 150 years ago.

I'm back in bed, seething in my morphine- and filth-induced rage, and have yet to speak to my surgeon. The cocky young surgery resident who assisted in my operation walks past the door with a young woman in scrubs. At least I think it is him; I can't see without my glasses on. He stops, looks in, and gives me a double thumbs-up sign like the Fonz and says, "Heyyyy," then he keeps walking. Seriously?

This is the same resident who, immediately following my surgery, went into the waiting area and told some random man all about my operation, without asking the guy

if he was my husband. Steve was sitting nearby and interrupted them. He explained who he was and the surgery
resident turned to my husband and repeated the information like he were pressing a tape recorder switch, without
apology. He told Steve and the random man that my surgery had gone well and, without elaborating, that they had
removed two or three lymph nodes during the procedure.

Before he is out of my very poor sight, I manage to get
his attention so that I can ask him why they removed some
of my lymph nodes. I'm worried that they saw something
they didn't like in there. He walks into the room pelvis
first, and the only explanation he gives about the lymph
nodes is, "Yeah, we do that sometimes." He has no idea
that I am a veterinary surgical oncologist or that I have
likely done this procedure many more times than he has.
He is a cocky little shit training to be a cocky big shit. I
know surgeons and residents like this, even in my doggie surgery world; some forget that they are dog doctors
and think they are God doctors. Dr. Fonz needs a major
smackdown, and I hope that one of the surgeons training
him is going to give it to him.

I'm alone again, but I do have my iPhone. It's my salva-
tion. I decide to bust out a text to some friends so that they
know I am okay. I keep it to inner-circle friends because I
don't have a great filter at the best of times and I can tell
the morphine is affecting my mood. I am not sure what is
going to come out.

> Hi guys, group text (sorry) to say hi, I'm okay. On mor-
> phine, which is not as fun as hydromorphone. Last
> time I was euphoric; this time very grumpy. The surgery

resident who just came to talk to me is a douche-tard.
They took a couple of nodes this time, which was not
the plan so am a bit stressed. Hopefully my surgeon is
coming soon to explain it to me. (Surg resident was clueless about this has no idea why they took nodes and was
patronizing and talked to me like I was a child.) Also,
the guy across hall with no legs is cranking volume on
his in-room documentaries for his/my listening pleasure
and I can't sleep but you can't tell a guy with no legs to
think of others. No legs card trumps thyroid cancer card,
every time. But I'm okay, really.

Love you guys,
X

My mood is pretty bad. I wish I could make it stop. I grab my iPad and do a quick search on PubMed of morphine and mood. I find information indicating that after being treated with morphine, patient satisfaction is low and side effects can include nausea, agitation, delirium, and hostility. Hydromorphone, on the other hand, is more likely to cause euphoria, good analgesia, and high patient satisfaction. I am definitely nauseous, possibly delerious, still in a bit of pain, and feeling rather hostile. My surgeon pops in and we discuss my lymph nodes in just a fraction more detail than I did with the cocky surgery resident. He says something like, "I did three completion thyroidecto-mies today, so I can't remember much about your lymph nodes." I do lots of surgeries in one day, too, and I can usu-ally remember each patient, especially when I am stand-ing in front of them or speaking to their owners. Anyway, bottom line is that some nodes came out but not for any particular reason. They are just out and that is the end of the explanation. The lymph node that I am concerned about, and wanted removed and biopsied is still sitting on my clavicle. I asked my surgeon before surgery if he would take it out and he looked at me with raised eyebrows and said, "We won't be doing that." At any rate, I guess I feel better having some random bits of lymphatic tissue being examined by a pathologist.

I am pretty frustrated that my request to remove the enlarged lymph node that has been bothering me all this time got shut down without discussion, especially because I know it would have taken about five minutes to remove it. I even fantasize that if I get a positive histopathology report or thyroid scan for spread of the thyroid cancer to my lymph nodes, I will re-enact the scene from *Good Will Hunting.* The one where Matt Damon gets Minnie Driver's phone number and slaps it dramatically against the window of the café where the rich snob guy who couldn't get Minnie's number is sitting, and yells, "Well, how do you like them apples?" Except that I am Matt Damon and my surgeon is the rich snob guy, and it is not Minnie Driver's phone number but the report saying the lymph nodes are positive (that part is highlighted in yellow for effect). It will probably never happen, because my nodes are expected to be negative, just like he says. Even if they were positive, I would need a copy of the report before the surgeon saw it and I would need to stumble upon him sitting in a café with his doctor friends, and there would need to be a window between us so that I could dramatically slap my report against it. Also, I would need a posse with me to witness the triumph and hilarity of the whole scene, and it wouldn't actually be that hilarious if my nodes are positive. It would be awful. I worry about it all the time.

I ask him if I can be switched from morphine to hydro-morphone and he says that it is not possible because hos-pital policy is to use morphine. I ask him if I can be put on ondansetron, the anti-nausea drug that I was on last time, because it worked perfectly. He says that hospital policy is to hold off on ondansetron until patients fail Gravol. They are saving money by putting me on morphine, which is in turn making me nauseous and angry, and then they are withholding the extremely effective anti-nausea drug, which is making me more angry. This is to save money. If the morphine is making me agitated, this cost-saving logic is making things worse. I start crying. I just want the same protocol that I had last time. Why can't I have it?

I imagine a group of non–medically trained hospital administrators in a boardroom somewhere, figuring out how much money they will save if they use morphine, not hydromorphone, and Gravol, not ondansetron. I am sure this looks great on their spreadsheet of tangible costs. However, I also suspect that the real costs are higher when hospitals use cheap drugs. It's a false economy. It's like buying cheap shampoo and then having to buy a lot more cheap hair products to compensate for how dull and life-less your hair looks. Or it's like buying cheap dog food that is full of fillers, so you have to feed your dog more than the expensive dog food (which ends up costing about the same, with the added bonus of a much higher volume of dog crap that you get to pick up). This hospital policy is the vicious cycle of bad hair. This hospital policy is the dog shit. How can it be less expensive to have nauseous, pain-ful, hostile patients, compared to comfortable, euphoric ones? How many more times will the first group call their nurses over to ask for help? How much more time does it take to deal with an agitated patient than a happy patient? What about patient satisfaction and the emotional toll that cancer surgery takes, let alone cancer surgery with a rough recovery? What about counting the intangible beans as well?

Between the morphine, the documentaries blasting next door, cleaning my own toilet, and the purple breast-flap fiasco, I am not having a restful recovery. It may not be fair, but I am focusing my morphine-induced anger on Samara. She is on her way out for the day, and in comes Rachel, the night nurse. Rachel is my sanity angel. She is lovely. She comes in and introduces herself, asks about my pain and if I need anything, gets me more ice, and assesses my neck incision and my face for signs of hypocalcemia (low calcium)—all in a span of about five minutes. I feel my whole body relax. I am so grateful. I ask her if I can switch to hydromorphone because the morphine is making me really unhappy, and somehow she achieves the impos-sible and makes it happen. When so much of the patient care is downloaded onto the nursing staff, a good nurse can make all the difference in the world.

The night is okay. I am much better on the hydromor-phone and I feel relatively peaceful. The next day I pray that Samara will not be here. She is not, but the alterna-tive is no better. Enter Lina, who comes in to check my vitals without a hello, good morning, how are you or an introduction. Unlike following my previous surgery, when my pain-control medication was given at regular intervals to coincide with the time when these medications would wear off, I now have to ask each time for pain medication and I am left to my own devices through most the day. Lina does the bare minimum and strives to do less. Any treatment or task she performs is done with a mixture of contempt and laziness. My blood calcium is monitored throughout the day and it turns out that my calcium is low. This is not devastating news on its own, since it is a known transient complication of the surgery, but it means that I can't go home today and will need to stay at least another twenty-four hours for treatment and monitoring. I am crushed.

I watch the clock and count down the time until Lina's twelve-hour shift ends. She does the same. At 8 p.m., Rachel, the Sanity Angel, walks into my room. She is cheerful, and she asks me how my day went as she assesses me. I am in tears again because I am so relieved that she is back, and I know that for the next twelve hours things will be okay.

The next morning Lina takes a blood sample and my blood pressure and temperature, chucks some pills at me, and leaves. I am given my oral thyroid medication and calcium at the same time. Later, I learn that when you take these medications at the same time, the calcium binds the thyroid medication and you don't absorb any of it. The head and neck surgery fellow comes in later and says that my calcium is a little better but still too low, and that they will have to check it again at noon and decide if I can go home. My Polish roommate is sprung today and I'm happy for her, but a little sad for myself that I am stuck here on my own. Even the blind legless man next door gets to go home. I see him with his family and he looks really happy. I am happy he gets to go home, too, because things just got a little quieter, but mostly I feel alone and sad. I just want to go home.

Lina takes my blood at noon and says it takes forty-five minutes to get results back. I wait. It is after 1:30 p.m. and I ring the buzzer, but no one comes. I'm so angry. I feel that I am not going to be able to control myself. It could be the morphine, the sleep deprivation, the second surgery, the cancer, the pain, the nausea, or just the mean nurses, but I can't take it any more. I head over to the nursing station and ask if they have my results back yet. Lina and the other nurses look up from their Facebook pages and just stare at me. I head back to bed. Another forty-five minutes goes by and Lina comes in with a script for my medications and a tiny strip of paper with the single post-operative instruction to call my surgeon's office on Monday. My calcium is the same as it was this morning. It is unclear to me whether or not this means that I should remain in the hospital. It is hard to tell which way it is going to go. It seems that I am leaving anyway. Thank God. Hypocalcemia can cause seizures if it is severe enough, and I am a little surprised that there is not a handout to explain this and some of the warning signs. I don't need the details, but most patients would. My clients have a long discharge appointment with me and go home with pages of written instructions; even then, the owners will usually have a long list of questions they need to discuss. Lina takes out my IV and I pack up to leave. I'm so angry that I can't even look at or speak to the gaggle of nurses as I walk past the nursing station. One of them says goodbye quietly, but it's too late. I'm already gone.

I text my friends again on the way home:

Hi all ☺ Just got discharged from the hospital/Ft. Knox. Not a banner morning. ☹ Whoever says the care at this hospital is amazing has obviously never met Lina. Calcium still a bit low and may have felt a secret facial twitch (shhhh!) but rolling the dice at home with the Vitamin D & Tums. Needed out.

X

ADMITTING VETERINARY PATIENTS FOR surgery is an art. You need to go over the client's goals and expectations and make a plan. You also have to go over the potential complications, because they are part of doing surgery. We do everything we can to minimize the possibility, but even with simple surgeries, the risk is never zero. I always go over everything verbally, but most owners are in a bit of a state when we have this conversation. The complications are therefore also written down and the clients have to sign the form to acknowledge that they understand the risks. This doesn't guarantee that people really understand what they're signing or even that they can read (I recently learned that 30 to 40 percent of Canadian adults have low literacy skills, so you can't assume anything). All we can do is our best and hope that if people don't fully understand the risks, at least they trust us and know we are honest and working in their pet's best interest.

There are varying degrees of written disclaimers that
veterinarians employ. I once worked with a veterinarian
who was a lawyer before becoming a vet. Without identify-
ing said veterinarian, I will say that his/her client consent
forms were filled with every conceivable and sometimes
inconceivable complication that could occur, and always
pre-empted by the phrase "Complications include, but are
not limited to..." It drove me crazy. It felt like an exercise in covering your ass. It felt sterile. It felt aggressive
and adversarial rather than caring. It felt like one of those
cheesy commercials for Viagra that starts out with a throaty
voice-over and an unreasonably good-looking older couple
who appear to be frisky, happy, flirty, and intimate and
have more libido than I have ever had, but ends with an
Alvin the Chipmunk voice-over quickly and cheerfully list-
ing off every imaginable risk: "complications include but
are not limited to back pain; diarrhea; dizziness; headache;
joint pain; skin rash; stomachache; stuffy nose; redness;
burning or swelling of the eye; inability to urinate; blurred
vision; chest pain; shortness of breath; prolonged, painful,
or inappropriate erection; severe pain; and death; in addi-
tion to which sexual intercourse has been reported to lead
to pregnancy..."

I think this litigious approach takes away from the
magic. One of my greatest mentors was at the other end
of the spectrum; he used to talk to clients and give it to
them straight. He was the best, and would do his best,
but sometimes shit happens. He probably even said that
to clients, because he was the kind of guy who could say
"shit happens" to clients and they would love him more
for it. He would spend a lot of time talking to his clients

and explaining the procedure and the risks, but he could not be asked to write out all the complications in a charade of covering his ass. He used to get out the necessary forms and hand them to clients to sign and say, "This one says that I'm not going to lie to you, and this one says that you are going to pay your bill." His typical admission form for patients coming in for limb-sparing surgery would just say "limb spare," the cost, and nothing else. This procedure has one of the highest complication rates in veterinary medicine, with a 40 percent infection rate, risk of implant failure, risk of local recurrence... and the list goes on. There is no doubt that he looked all of his clients in the eye, told them all of the risks, and ensured that they understood. He is a legend.

My approach to this kind of paperwork is somewhere in the middle. I would prefer to be more like my mentor, but the reality is that sometimes clients will turn on you when things have not gone their way, and I am not him. He is untouchable. Clients can have selective hearing or memories sometimes, and if you don't write down what you have said, it never happened. If things start going south, clients will always say that they wouldn't have opted for surgery if they had known things were going to go south. I think that is pretty obvious. That's the way life goes. You wouldn't take a job if you knew that your favourite mentor and colleague was going to die suddenly six months later and leave you working with an utter sociopath. You wouldn't get married if you knew that your spouse was going to stop loving you one day. You wouldn't buy a house if you knew that the market was about to crash. You wouldn't give your whole heart to a dog if you knew that he would die one day.

I try to take a straightforward, honest approach. I am blunt about the disease and the risks, but I try to soften this with my sense of humour and the fact that there are a lot of options. I go over the complications and then I concede to the world I live in and write it all down so the client can acknowledge that they have understood the risks by signing the form.

Most of the complaints veterinarians receive are related to money and complications, and the fact that complications cost money. Canadian pet owners struggle with the cost of veterinary care more than Americans do. They are not used to receiving a big bill for health care and have no idea what their own health care costs. They think that their own health care is free. Some of them even suggest that their pet's health care should also be covered by the Government of Canada.

A very compassionate and wealthy Canadian donor, whom I was touring around our hospital, asked me quite earnestly, "What do people do if they can't afford treatment for their pets?" It was as if this had never occurred to her before. She was utterly horrified to learn that some people cannot and do not treat their pets for financial reasons. I wondered if I should remind her that there are also people who can't afford medical and dental care for themselves or other specialty items, like food and clothing.

Specialization in veterinary medicine just exacerbates the money problem. The more advanced the care, the more it is going to cost. None of this occurred to me when I decided that I wanted to specialize in small animal surgery. It was unceremoniously pointed out to me by one of my hippie friends when I told him that I wanted to do a surgery residency: "So, you are going to spend your career taking care of rich people's animals?" This is possibly one of the meanest things that anyone has ever said to me. It also happens to be true. My friend ended up becoming an engineer and working for an oil company, so I am not sure he gets to keep his moral high ground, but this comment has stuck with me and still bothers me two decades later.

Sasha was a miniature poodle heiress. I met her after she developed a neurological abnormality. Her face looked asymmetrical to the owners, and they were not the type of clients to let anything wait. They rushed her to the emergency room and then to a veterinary neurologist. Sasha's clinical signs were mild and were considered likely to resolve. It was suggested that an MRI could be done if she did not improve. She improved, but the owners went ahead with the MRI anyway. The MRI revealed a surprising finding. Sasha had a bone tumour arising from her skull. It was almost impossible to detect the mass from the outside because it was growing down into her frontal sinus. Although the symptoms she was originally brought in for were probably not related to the mass, it was serendipitous that her owners were so wealthy that they didn't need to think twice about spending $2,500 on an MRI.

Once the diagnosis of a skull mass was made, Sasha's owners immediately sprang into action. The mass was biopsied and the results came back as a type of bone tumour called an MLO (multilobular osteochondroma), which usually has a good prognosis when it is treated with surgery. Sasha was referred to our oncology service to go over options. Surgery would offer the best chance of a cure but also had the greatest potential for complications, including severe blood loss and even death. Radiation would give us control of the tumour for a period of months to a year, but it would be unlikely to cure the cancer, and Sasha's owners might be faced with the same decision about taking her to surgery a year from then. They contemplated radiation, but they would have to go to the States to get this done because it was a very specialized type of radiation. I told the owner that the cost of treatment was around $6,000 and he told me that was a fraction of the cost of the private jet he would use to take her there.

The owners were leaning toward surgery. They wanted the best chance for Sasha. The surgery she needed is called a craniectomy, in which the affected portion of the skull and a cuff of normal bone surrounding it are removed. We went over the risks of the procedure in detail, which include permanent brain damage, severe hemorrhage, and death. Sasha's owners found talking about the complications difficult and they went very quiet for a while. One of her owners then said that she found the conversation sobering. That was the idea.

As veterinarians, we never intend to scare owners, but we do want to make sure they understand the risks. Money can't prevent these complications. We always do our best, regardless of how much money the owners have, but sometimes shit happens. The reality is that having deep pockets makes complication management easier. Complications from surgery are costly, hard to quote for, and generate a tremendous amount of stress for the client, the veterinarian and, of course, the patient. Most veterinarians have an unhealthy tendency to blame themselves or question if they did anything wrong. Unfortunately, many clients can be just as quick to try to assign blame. If Sasha needed to be on a ventilator post-operatively, required multiple blood transfusions, or had a prolonged hospital stay for any reason, these owners would be able to afford the care. Veterinary critical care has become so advanced that sometimes it is the cost to treat the patient per day, rather than the disease process itself, that can kill a critically ill patient, meaning that even some patients who are very ill can recover if their owners can afford the care.

Sasha's owners were in a fortunate position where money was no issue. Sasha's surgery was going to cost anywhere from $6,000 to $10,000 depending on the complications—with no guarantees. She had her surgery, and it could not have gone more perfectly. The mass came out without incident and she didn't even require a blood tranfusion, which is a feat for a dog her size. Her recovery was smooth and she was sitting up in her cage just a few hours after surgery. Her owners visited the day after surgery and she looked so normal to them that they wanted to take her home. They hated being apart from Sasha. We were outside with them during their visit and they even showed me how Sasha recognized their Rolls in the parking lot and wanted to hop in and go back home. Unfortunately, I had to tell them that Sasha needed to stay another night to be sure that she didn't experience any complications, such as bleeding or seizures.

The three of us stood beside their Rolls, arguing gently and joking with each other about whether or not she really needed to stay. It was light-hearted, but they kept pushing me to send Sasha home, and even casually threw out the suggestion that I would liable if something happened to her in the hospital after I refused to send her home. That almost worked, but despite feeling a bit concerned that I could be sued, bought, and sold if something did happen to her, I stuck to my guns and kept her for one more night of monitoring. I suspect that *no* is not a word Sasha's owners have heard very often.

Sasha continued to have a better than average recovery and was eating her homemade lamb chunks and wagging her tail the next morning. She went home that afternoon. Her final bill was only $4,200. I was happy not to be over quote, but it was ironic that I would end up $1,800 below the low end of the estimate for the family that needed a break the least. For some clients, even going a few hundred dollars over quote can be upsetting, because they've only budgeted for the initial quote. It is difficult to be as precise as we want to be at predicting the final bill. There are just too many variables.

At Sasha's discharge, her owners presented us with a thank-you card and headed out the door. The card contained a $50,000 cheque to support our cancer centre. There was no ceremony to this gift, no strings attached, and they didn't wait around to be sucked up to, thanked, or flattered. They were simply levelling the playing field and paying what they could to save a family member who is priceless.

Not everyone can afford anything beyond basic veterinary care for their pets. For some pet owners, no matter how they budget, they just can't do it. For others, it is a matter of priorities. All I care about is that animals are treated humanely and that they do not suffer. What people decide to spend on their pets is nobody's business but their own.

Here are the top ten outrageous comments that I hear about the cost of veterinary care:

1. A bullet costs only ninety-nine cents.

2. Just go to the shelter and get a new (healthy) dog.

3. If you (the vet) really loved animals, you would take care of them for free.

4. You should spend the money on starving children instead of fixing a dog.

5. It's only a dog.

6. It's only a cat.

7. Veterinarians must all be rich. *(I can assure you, we are not.)*

8. I have spent so much money here, I probably own a wing of this hospital. *(But not really.)*

9. Can I get pet insurance now that will cover this? *(No, because that is called fraud.)*

10. Why would anyone spend so much money on a dog? *(Invalidating my whole career.)*

Maybe it is just jealousy that makes people so vicious: jealousy about not understanding why a dog is worth so

much more than a ninety-nine-cent bullet, why someone would go to such lengths for a dog. If you have ever
been lucky enough to let a dog into your heart, you will
understand.

THE DAY TSOTSI DIED, I would have paid anything to save
him. Leading up to that day, if you had asked me to name
the one thing I couldn't live without, I would have said
Tsotsi. He was my golden retriever–border collie cross
who had loved me all through veterinary school. He had
the best qualities of both breeds and he was *that* dog, the
one my clients are always telling me about. The soulmate
dog that you might only be lucky enough to have once in
your lifetime. He was so smart. I trained him to sit at every
curb until he was released to cross the road. I thought this
would keep him safe. I walked him off-leash all over Saskatoon, and he always stuck by me and stopped abruptly
at every curb to wait for me. It was adorable.

When Tsotsi was nine, Steve and I were living in Guelph
during my surgery residency. My husband took Tsotsi and
Molly (our other dog) for a walk in an off-leash area.
Somehow Tsotsi got into a ravine near the parking lot,
crossed under the road through a large pipe, and popped
up on the other side. I wasn't there, but I imagine that
he was sitting on the other side of the road, waiting to
be released, because that is what he always did. My husband called him, with his back to the road, not realizing
that Tsotsi was on the other side. Tsotsi, always obedi-
ent, crossed the road. Steve turned around when he heard
a loud thud behind him and saw the truck drive off. He

gathered up my broken dog and rushed him to the hospital where I was working. When he arrived, I was just coming out of surgery and setting up one of my patients in the ICU. I was in a great mood, which was interrupted by a man yelling in the ICU triage area.

I went over to see what was going on, not realizing that the yelling man was Steve and that the lifeless dog in his arms was my dog—my heart. I called for help. My friends and colleagues sprang into action, but it was hopeless. They started CPR, on Tsotsi as I stood there watching; I was powerless and hysterical. They cracked his chest to start open CPR, and litres of blood poured out of him. One of the residents went to get a bag of blood to start a transfusion. The head of the ICU touched her shoulder and told her quietly to get an expired bag. I heard her, and I knew what she meant—they needed to go through the motions of trying to resuscitate Tsotsi to make me feel like they had tried, but his heart had ruptured, his entire blood volume was in his chest, and it was hopeless. My beautiful dog was dead. They shouldn't waste a good bag of blood on him. It wasn't worth it.

I was just a resident, so I didn't have a lot of money, but I would have done anything in that moment to revive him. I would have remortgaged the house, sold my truck, sold my kidney, sold my body, anything, so that he could live. My soulmate dog and my most faithful companion for the past nine years was gone. I wailed over his body for an indeterminate period of time until I was shuffled home. There, I wailed so hard and loud and crazy that my husband closed all the windows because he thought someone might call the police and report a domestic.

Maybe it was the shock factor—or the fact that it was so graphic—but standing in the ICU, watching my beautiful dog's ruptured heart bleed and seeing him die in front of me, remains one of the worst days of my life. I will never shake the image of his open chest and the dark red blood pouring over his soft golden fur. I can still hear the splattering sound of his blood hitting the floor. Maybe some people might think this means that I have had a relatively great life, but pain isn't relative. Horrific experiences are not comparable. Tsotsi taught me about intense love and loss, and the deep hole a dog can rip in your heart.

I AM STILL NOT having a great recovery from my second surgery. The two weeks since surgery have been pretty horrible. I think that I was telling myself to keep it together until this surgery. But as soon as it was over, everything seemed to unravel. I unravelled. I had been on a see-saw of over- and under-reaction, and after my surgery I lost the balance. My thyroid cancer is a middle ground of happy disaster and sad relief. Happy disaster because I am supposed to be happy about my good cancer, and sad relief because I'm relieved that I advocated for myself, but it has taken its toll. My anger was always brewing under the surface, but the narcotics and the sleep deprivation unleashed it. There are a few things that I need to get off my chest. I am full to the brim with the self-righteous wrath of a cancer survivor. There are so many easy targets: the patronizing doctors, the eye-rolling nurses, the apathetic care workers, smokers (just in general, they make me so mad! Why is anyone still smoking? And why is it still legal? Why don't smokers have to pay more for medical insurance? Why would you do something to yourself that you know will give you cancer?), and our inefficient health care system.

I feel the wrath bubble up sometimes when I least expect it. I have just received a fundraising letter from the hospital where I had my second surgery. The hospital to which I have just sent a letter, complaining about the nursing care I received and their ill-conceived cost-saving medication policies. There doesn't seem to be any coordination between the patient relations department and the development department. The mere sight of the envelope makes me feel wrath. It is blue, with fluffy clouds. "It is when we are at our weakest that we find our greatest strength" is written across the front in an inspirational font — so clichéd, lame, and transparent. It might as well say, "It is when you are at your weakest that we find you will donate the most money," or "If things don't go well for you, remember us in your will."

Inside, more lack of coordination, this time not with my desire to donate but with my disease. The letter is all about a young woman who almost died on her wedding day and then received a mechanical heart, and later a transplant, and now has a new life. It's not even about cancer. Can't they at least get that straight? Cancer patients should get a cancer story and heart patients should get a heart disease story. I wasn't touched by heart disease. I was touched by cancer. Inside the envelope—for my enjoyment—are ten ugly Christmas cards on cheap stock that I will never use. I wish they hadn't sent me the cards and had instead donated the money used to create this cheap swag to themselves.

In a later fundraising campaign, the hospital sent me a letter that was full of stickers with pictures of the ribbons for all types of cancer, only thyroid cancer wasn't one of them. The only sticker that applied to me was the blank ribbon that said "other" underneath it, with instructions to fill in my own cancer colour. Wow, thanks. I feel very special. I'm an "other cancer" survivor. I will stick this sticker on something with pride. Your extremely personal gift has overwhelmed me with a desire to donate to your hospital.

Maybe I am just a little cancer-irritable right now, but I'm also pretty pissed off at Statistics Canada. They won't leave me alone. Statistics Canada and its aggressive task force have randomly selected me as a participant for a survey on the environment, and are stalking me.

I have managed to avoid dealing with this for months, but one day, a brilliant young surveyor finally captures me on my cellphone. I don't realize that it is Stats Canada until it is too late, because they have never called my cellphone before. I can hear that the guy on the other end of the phone is gleeful that he has me. He explains that they would like me to participate in their survey, but that it is not mandatory. I interrupt.

"Excuse me, if this is not mandatory, then I do not wish to participate."

He is not happy with this answer. "Can I ask why not?"

"Because I am not feeling well."

Without a pause or a breath, he begins to tell me how important it is that I participate in this survey. I am trying to be polite.

"Look, I'm trying to be polite. Please can you just

accept that I don't wish to participate because I am not feeling well?"

No, he can't. My opinion on the environment appears to be highly sought after, for some inexplicable reason. He doesn't even try to hide the fact that he is mad. His voice quickly takes on a mocking, sarcastic tone: "So you want me to make a note that you refuse to participate in the survey because you are not feeling well today?"

Okay, that's it, here comes the C-card. Don't say I didn't warn you, bitch.

"I don't want to participate because I have not been feeling well for the past six months because I have cancer and I'm a little busy dealing with that."

He wasn't expecting this response. "Oh, okay, I'll make a note of that in your file."

He made me do it. It's the only time I have pulled the C-card like that. You would think that would have been enough to make the calls stop, but Statistics Canada is rabid and relentless. Six days later, the phone calls start again. I think I need a restraining order.

Am I really just mad because I have cancer? I don't think so; that would be like getting mad at a hurricane or a tornado. It's just nature. I did poke around for a while to see if there was something I could blame, a risk factor that I could focus on and obsess about, but for me, there was nothing. I have no Chernobyl. It's just genetics. My genetics. It is not really anything to get mad about. And everyone says it's good cancer. It's so good.

I am not mad at my cancer. It is more the navigation through this treatable and curable cancer that has caused all the wrath.

There has been a letting go, too. I think that I am starting to lose my edge, in a good way. This bitch is tired and
it's hard to be mad all the time. The fighting and advocacy
wears you down. I have found a way not to go into fight-
or-flight mode and to just stay put where I am. I have found
the peace in not reacting—there is always time to freak
out later if you still care. Cancer has taught me to have
perspective on anger; it helps me decide when the wrath is
worthwhile and when to see it for what it is: a sin against
myself.

I THOUGHT ABOUT NORTH a lot when I was trying to stay positive about my own cancer.

North had a big problem with his nose, but everything else in his life was great. He had lived a long and perfect life with his loving owner. North went to Starbucks for coffee-and-cookie dates, and he hiked five to six kilometres on the Bruce Trail every day. Wherever his owner went, North went, too. There was just this thing with his nose.

It started out as a small ulcerated area in his left nostril. It looked like a sore, but it wasn't healing and was getting bigger. I think it was pretty painful, but he would never let anyone know it. The other dog in his family would not leave his nose alone. She kept following him, sniffing and licking his nose and trying to get someone's attention. North was handsome and dignified. He was a thirteen-and-a-half-year-old golden retriever. He went to see his family veterinarian, who biopsied the abnormal area in his nostril. It came back as a squamous cell carcinoma, an aggressive cancer that originates from the tissue that lines the nose or mouth. This is what brought North to me.

North had a light gold face, a white muzzle, dark eyes, and a dark nose. Except for the obvious, he was in perfect health. The tumour had not spread beyond his nose and was unlikely to do so. With surgery, he could be cured, which was all good news. The bad news was that no matter what happened, he was going to lose his nose—to either the tumour or the surgery. We needed to cut off his nose to save his face.

His owner took the news well. She was brave and had a great sense of humour. Not that any of it was funny, but sometimes you have to look for the humour in the tragedy. The cancer was aggressive and disfiguring. The surgery would be aggressive and disfiguring. No one wants to sign up their dog for the aggressive and disfiguring surgery plan, but that was what it was going to take to cure North's cancer.

The day that North came back for his surgery, his owner brought me a collage of pictures of his face throughout his life. She wanted me to see how nice his nose was before his nasal tumour and his surgeon (me) came along. He did have a great nose.

We had to remove the cute black part of his nose (the entire nasal planum). To try to make it look a little better, and to prevent anyone from being able to look inside his nasal cavity like he was a *Star Wars* character, his upper lip was used to help reconstruct the defect. I called the owner after surgery and explained that North was doing fine and recovering in ICU. I told her that he now looked like a cross between a golden retriever and a pug, so I was going to start calling him a guggle. Not every owner would find this amusing, but I knew that she would. She didn't care what he looked like, as long as he was comfortable and the tumour was gone for good. He recovered well and by the next morning he was smiling and showing off his funny new face.

North's cancer was cured, so he didn't need to come back for medical appointments or any further treatment, but I received regular email updates from his owner, usually in the form of a Smilebox photo montage of North that was set to music and made me cry every time. She thought he felt better now that the tumour was gone and that he had more energy. With very stoic patients, sometimes we can only diagnose pain or discomfort in retrospect, when we have removed it or treated its source. North continued to hike the Bruce Trail and frequent Starbucks. When he was at the park, the other dog owners didn't ask her, "What happened to your dog?" They asked, "What breed is that?" His owner always answered very seriously that he was a cancer-free breed. You know, a guggle.

North lived for another eighteen months. His owner had to let him go because of mobility issues and prostatic disease, none of which were related to his nasal cancer diagnosis. North's veterinarian euthanized him when he was fifteen. A success story, to be sure, but his owner's heart still broke on his last day. The night before they put him down, the entire family got together and ate barbequed steaks and rasberry ice cream for desert. Nobody was particularly hungry, including North, but he appreciated the menu and the effort. His owner lay beside him all night, not sleeping, wishing for time to slow down and cursing the dawn. The next morning, she took him for a walk in one of his favourite parks and to Starbucks for coffee and a cookie. Then she took him to her family veterinarian and held him until his last breath.

If you lose your nose to cancer and you are a dog, you can still be cute. "He is so ugly he is cute" is something that is said only about animals. If a person loses his nose to cancer, the social implications are devastating. During my residency, there was a man I used to see downtown who had lost his entire nose to cancer. I would see him walking around with a small piece of gauze taped over his nose holes. On windy days, the gauze would blow up and you could see in. Without a nose, every social interaction is unkind. Wearing glasses is impossible. Getting a job is difficult. Your voice sounds weird. It sounds nasally, which is counterintuitive and makes no sense. People can't help themselves: they stare. I have stared. He couldn't afford a prosthesis, so a social worker in our community raised money to get a prosthetic nose made for him. The story was in the local paper, and he suddenly looked happy in the accompanying photos. How can a rubber nose make so much difference to how we treat a man? Are we really that shallow? Why can't we just laugh off the new, cancer-free noseless look for a man the way we could for North?

Veterinary patients don't care as much about missing body parts and they are less vulnerable to being judged if they look strange. Even if they are being judged, they don't know that they are being judged. All the judging and shame is human. Being a veterinary (and I assume human) surgical oncologist is about knowing the limits. To do this job, you need a combination of humour, confidence, training, compassion, swagger, creativity, and surgical bravado. In short, you need mojo. Without mojo, you are sunk.

A surgeon with no mojo will tell a client, "Your dog has a sarcoma. This tumour needs a big surgery to remove it all. We can do that, but it will be aggressive and disfiguring. We will probably need to do a blood transfusion and your dog could bleed to death. Your dog might not make it through surgery and it is going to be really expensive." A surgeon with mojo will say, "Your dog has a sarcoma. This is an aggressive tumour that is disfiguring. We have a chance to cure your dog, but it requires a big surgery to make sure we get it all. Your dog will not look normal after surgery, but when his hair grows in, he will look okay and you will get used to it. There are some risks that include bleeding, tumour recurrence in the future, anesthetic complications, and even death. I will give you a quote to tell you what it is going to cost." The difference is subtle, but crucial for someone who is considering handing their dog over for surgery.

Mambo's owners told me that they agreed to his surgery because I seemed so confident; I guess that was the mojo. Mambo's was a case that required a lot of mojo. Mambo was a yellow lab and a Seeing-Eye-dog-school dropout. I suspect that his inability to sit still and his consuming passion for people, doughnuts, and ice cream were factors that held him back from his original career path. He was actually rejected twice as a Seeing Eye dog and was adopted by his family when he was two years old. What Mambo lacked in discipline and focus in his previous vocation, he made up for with endless energy and wild, crazy love. When his adoptive family went to meet him for the first time, he came bounding out of the cage and bowled them over, tail spinning. Mowing people down as a form of greeting and free-spiritedness are not ideal traits in a Seeing Eye dog, but it was love at first sight for the whole family, and Mambo went home with them that day.

At only four years of age, Mambo developed a sarcoma around his eye. His eye and the tumour were removed at another hospital and he was referred to ours for radiation. Tumour cells had been left behind after his first surgery, and just three weeks later, the mass was back and filling his now empty eye socket; an MRI confirmed it. There was too much tumour for radiation to be effective, so we recommended a second surgery. This time, the surgery would be radical. In surgical oncology terms, *radical* means removal of an entire anatomic segment. When I describe radical surgery to my students, I tell them that *radical* is another word for *awesome*, because we can cure some of these patients with radical surgery, and that is awesome. For Mambo, this would mean removing his eye socket, the skin around the eye, part of his skull, and part of his upper jaw. There were definitely some major risks with the surgery, but without it there was no risk, just the certainty that he would die—and soon.

Mambo's family consisted of a couple in their fifties and their daughter, who was a young adult. Mambo was the heart and soul of the family and the glue that held them together. I couldn't tell who Mambo's primary owner was, because they all loved him so much and were all so invested in his care. Each had their own way of trying to make the decision about the surgery. The daughter cried every night and the dad gathered as much information as he could, asking more and more questions every time we spoke. The mom thought the fact that the song "Mambo Italiano" was on the radio a lot in a pizza commercial was a sign that they should go ahead. You couldn't help but sing that song to him when you saw him. Mambo's entire hind end swivelled when he wagged his tail, and it definitely looked like his own interpretation of his namesake song. Sometimes a song on the radio is all it takes to make a big decision, to tell you what you already know. The owners put their trust in me and gave me a privilege that I will never take for granted, no matter how many surgeries I do. We took Mambo to surgery.

It was a long surgery, taking several hours, but it was a success. The surgeon may be the one with the mojo and the glory, but a big surgery like this is a huge team effort. It takes the expertise of veterinary anesthesiologists, criticalists, radiologists, medical oncologists, technicians, and a great facility to make it happen. Everyone works together for a successful outcome and, as my mentor used to tell me, the patient is the one that takes all the risk.

Mambo recovered in our ICU on a fine cocktail of three different pain medications, since big surgeries also require big pain relief. The defect created by the surgery required a skin flap for reconstruction, which was harvested from his neck. I thought he looked fantastic. His owner thought he looked like a Frankendog, and she burst into tears when she saw him. He was pretty drugged, but even through his opioid haze, he recognized her and showed her that his tail was still working, and that he was going to be okay.

About a week after surgery, the tip of the skin flap used on Mambo's face turned black and died; he needed two revision procedures to heal completely. Eventually, he ended up with a large swath of long neck hair across the side of his otherwise smooth face, covering the site where his left eye and the tumour had been. It looked like a cross between a mohawk, a bathmat, and a Phantom of the Opera mask. It was a great look for him and it really just added to his carefree nature and wild sense of personal style.

We recommended chemotherapy for Mambo after his surgery because the tumour type, a high-grade osteo-sarcoma, had a high chance of metastasizing. We had to delay the chemotherapy until he had completely healed from his revision surgeries, which made his owners nervous. They had already seen how fast this tumour could recur. Mambo's first chemotherapy dose did not go well. He was nauseous and weak, and he didn't want to eat. Mambo not wanting to eat is like other dogs not wanting to breathe. This is a dog who would recognize every Tim Hortons and his favourite ice cream shop as he passed by in the car and would protest emphatically if he did not get to stop for doughnuts or a kiddie cone. All that Seeing Eye dog training was not wasted on Mambo. He had skills.

Mambo had to be hospitalized for a day for supportive care. Once he recovered, we adjusted his chemotherapy regimen a bit and the rest of his treatments were uneventful. After this incident, the only call we received from his owners during his course of chemotherapy was to ask us if they should be worried that Mambo had eaten an entire carrot cake that had been sitting on the counter. He was back to chasing tractors, swimming in the forbidden pond, and eating things that he shouldn't eat. On Mambo's fifth birthday, after he had finished all his treatments and was back to being a dog, Mambo and his owners came to visit us at the hospital and brought us a huge birthday cake. Carrot cake, of course—Mambo's favourite.

Mambo was in remission for sixteen months. When he came out of remission, the tumour came back with a vengeance; we saw evidence of tumour regrowth along the incisions where the tumour had been, and metastasis in his lungs. We tried a new type of chemotherapy and his owners reached for holistic solutions for a few weeks, but ultimately, his cancer was back and there was nothing more we could do. He stopped eating again, and the owners knew what that meant. They euthanized him at our hospital. He went peacefully, with his head resting on his favourite stuffed bunny pillow and his owners rubbing his belly as they all cried and said goodbye.

Is sixteen months a long time or a short time? Is it worth the money and the morbidity? Was the treatment for him or for his family? Is it selfish to want him to live, or would a dog want to live, too, if we could ask him? Is living with cancer for sixteen months better than dying of it in a few weeks? These are questions that don't have answers. Trying to generate a concrete answer does a disservice to our clients and our patients. Ultimately, are we just buying time? Yes, I think that is all that any of us are doing when we treat cancer. Can these patients handle it? Yes, better than most human patients do. Mambo's and North's owners said they would do it all again, and that is enough for me. Dogs don't despair that they don't look perfect or that they have just had surgery. They stay in the moment, finding joy in the doughnuts and cookies (which I am not advocating), long walks, and swims with their owners— they have more mojo than I could ever hope to have.

IT'S TIME FOR MY three-week post-op appointment with my surgeon. I am doing okay, much better, really. I am recovering from the physical and emotional havoc of surgery. I'm healing well and removed my own sutures two weeks ago. My voice is fine, too, so no worries about the nerves to my larynx. I'm seeing my surgeon today anyway. He comes in and launches into the histopathology report from my completion thyroidectomy.

The normal side that was just removed has multiple microcarcinomas in it that are up to 2 millimetres in size, and the nodes he biopsied are clear. Microcarcinomas? Multiple tiny tumours? Huh? Can we back up a second? He glossed over the multiple microcarcinomas part so quickly that I almost missed it. Apparently, these tiny specklings of cancer are found in 30 percent of thyroid cancer patients, and nobody is concerned but me. Despite being told that this is normal, or at least cancer-normal, I am concerned that this genetic mistake was able to repeat itself over and over again in my thyroid gland. It makes me wonder what has been going on in there. I worry that my thyroid gland—possibly my whole body—is a cancer factory. Veterinarians call golden retrievers cancer factories sometimes, because they have been inbred for their beauty and lovely temperament and, as an unfortunate consequence, are genetically predisposed to multiple forms of cancer. Am I basically a golden retriever now? What is my thyroid gland's problem?

My surgeon talks to me about the next steps, which might include potential radioactive iodine treatment to ablate any remaining thyroid tissue. I can tell that he doesn't think I should do it. I am in a grey zone as far as this decision goes, but he is trying to steer me over to his way of thinking. He tells me about the guidelines he follows, which recommend radioactive iodine for all patients with tumours that are 4 centimetres or larger. Other sources recommend that radioactive iodine ablation be performed for all carcinomas that are larger than 2 centimetres. My tumour was 3.8 centimetres on ultrasound and 3.2 centimetres after being fixed in formalin once it was removed. The studies that have been used to come up with this size guideline are sometimes based on ultrasound measurement and sometimes based on formalin-fixed tissue. There is no consensus for masses that are 2 to 4 centimetres. We have been over this before, and I have done my own research on whether or not radioactive iodine is advisable. But whichever way you look at it, there doesn't seem to be any accounting for a mass that pops out of nowhere and grows quickly.

My surgeon's opinion is based on the fact that there is no survival advantage to radioactive iodine, but he does say that an increase in recurrence is more likely if you don't get radioactive iodine. I want to know that I have done everything I can to prevent recurrence. I want to know that I can monitor for recurrence easily, through a blood test. If you are not treated with radioactive iodine, those blood test results can be equivocal.

I don't want equivocal. I just want to be done. I want to know what is happening in the lymph nodes in my neck. The plump ones that I can feel and see are bigger than normal. They ache, but I can't tell if it is all in my head. He feels my resistance to the "wait and see" approach and then shrugs it off, saying that it is not up to him anyway— the radiation oncologist that he referred me to will help me decide. End of discussion.

He sends me to the lab for some blood work to check my thyroid levels. I am done with everything in about ten minutes. I'm supposed to come back in three or six months and see him or the radiation oncologist or the endocrinologist or someone. Not sure. I put some sort of reminder in my phone to go see someone in three months. I ask him who is in charge of my case now and he says basically everyone (i.e., no one).

I head to the lab. To get there, you have to cross the food court, which looks like an unremarkable mall food court, except that it's in a hospital. These fast food restaurants sit exactly below the cardiac institute. Cardiologists, dietitians, and nurses are likely counselling their patients not to eat this crappy, salty, fatty food at the very same moment that I cross the food court underneath them. You can pick up a burger and fries on the way to the lab to get your skyrocketing cholesterol checked. How convenient. Then, on your way out, you can drop by the pharmacy to pick up some Lipitor and anti-hypertension medications to drive down your cholesterol and blood pressure. It is one-stop shopping.

Now there is nothing to do but wait until my appointment with the radiation oncologist, which is five weeks from now and was booked three weeks ago, at the time of my second surgery. I start to obsess about the date and the fact that I have to wait five weeks. I made a few sad attempts to get my appointment moved up by calling the radiation oncologist's assistant. She was nice, but there was no chance. I asked if I could be put on a waiting list, imagining that some people probably die waiting to get an appointment, so this might free up a spot, and she told me that she would make a note, which was probably a sticky note, because there was no formal waiting list. I even asked my surgeon for help. Apparently, he had just called the radiation oncologist about another thyroid cancer patient of his who had a much more aggressive form of thyroid carcinoma than mine. He couldn't get her moved up, so he said there was no way I would get in any sooner. He might as well have said, "She is *dying* and she has to wait, so you have to wait longer." I also cyberstalked the radiation oncologist for a while and considered sending him an email, hoping to make a connection. Some physicians really like veterinarians, so I thought it might help if I tried the "one medicine" angle. But I couldn't find his email and I doubt it would have helped anyway. I wait out the five weeks. Time flies when you're having cancer.

My radiation oncology appointment is at the sarcoma clinic. I am not completely confident that I am in the right place because the location was switched from the sarcoma clinic to the head and neck clinic and back to the sarcoma clinic during the time I waited for this appointment; the date changed once, too (pushed back three days). I check in. Without looking up, the receptionist asks me to put my blue hospital card in the Plexiglas box on the counter. Everyone in this room has cancer and is waiting to talk to someone about radiation. Some of them have bad cancer. I can tell. Is it too much to ask that the receptionist at the sarcoma clinic look up for a second and acknowledge me? Yes, it is. I drop the card in the box and sit down.

After about forty minutes, I am moved into an examination room. Twenty minutes later, a harried nurse comes in to tell me that she is so sorry about the wait and that they are running behind. I am shocked, not because I have been waiting for an hour, but because someone in this system finds the waiting unacceptable and seems to care.

The radiation oncologist finally enters. He is very nice. I tell him what I do and that I have a good understanding of radioactive iodine ablation and how it works. He goes over it all anyway, discussing the pros and cons of treatment with radioactive iodine. Radioactive iodine kills the thyroid tissue (cancerous and normal cells) but spares the rest of the cells in the body. Iodine is used to make thyroid hormone, so the only cells in the body that are able to absorb iodine are thyroid cells. Thyroid cells will transport iodine across their cell membranes and inside the cell to make thyroid hormone. You can manipulate these cells to avidly take the radioactive iodine inside, which kills the cells. It is supercool. Radioactive iodine is the Trojan Horse of cancer treatment.

In order to prepare for radioactive iodine, you need to have a high level of thyroid-stimulating hormone (TSH) in your body. You can achieve this either by taking a drug called Thyrogen (which is synthetic TSH) or by stopping all your thyroid medication for five to six weeks. If you don't have a thyroid gland and you stop taking thyroid medication, your body tries to stimulate your absent thyroid gland to get to work by making more TSH. Stopping all thyroid medication is called "going hypo" in the biz. Taking Thyrogen sounds like a lot more fun than going hypo, but it turns out that the only plant in the world that makes Thyrogen has just been shut down due to a contamination issue. This has resulted in a global shortage for an undetermined period of time. Of course it has. This means that I will be going hypo because it is the only option.

Going hypo sounds hard. The radiation oncologist says I will feel awful. He is kind and accommodating and lets me have a say in my health care decisions. In the end, I decide to do the radioactive iodine treatment. His nurse comes in and we set up a date. She explains the steps that will lead up to treatment: The first step is to switch from the long-acting thyroid medication that I am on to a short-acting thyroid medication called Cytomel. This gives your body time to get rid of the long-acting thyroid medication but allows you to feel somewhat normal (for the time being). Then you go off everything and feel very lethargic. A week before the treatment, you have to start a low-iodine diet. She gives me a handout and we fill in the dates for each step. It is all so reasonable. I feel I have turned a corner and gained some control of my disease and my life, all without having to fight.

After my appointment they ask me to drop in to the lab again (a now-routine stop). This time the blood work they want is not for me but for their tumour bank. The system has identified me as a study patient with an efficiency that I have not seen in the system until now. It is 4:10 p.m. and the lab closes at 5 p.m. I wait in line at the window. No one is there. While I am waiting, someone comes out the door after her shift and makes no attempt to alert her co-workers to the growing line of people at the window. She is off duty. A lab tech finally takes me back and looks at my requisition on the computer and tells me that she can't take my blood because they don't take blood for research after 4 p.m. She explains this to me as if it is my fault, my problem, and as if I care. If I hadn't waited for over an hour for my radiation appointment, I would have been right on time for her to stick a needle in my arm again. It's too bad I am going to miss out on that—I was looking forward to it. I roll down my sleeve and head out.

The next day, I am checking in with my endocrinologist. I am now his favourite patient and he makes a big fuss over me. Humility is good for our relationship. He bumps up my dose of thyroid medication by a minuscule amount, which is good, because I constantly feel like I am running out of gas. I am Sarah unplugged. Everything is slow in the world of endocrinology. Hopefully the increase in dose will help me to feel more energetic, but trying to find the right dose of thyroid medication is slow going. Doses are titrated and the effects are seen in weeks to months and then adjusted again until the fine-tuning is perfect and your dose is perfect and you feel perfect.

Everyone says that one day I will be back to normal; every thyroid anecdote ends positively. The usual story is someone telling me about their friend/aunt/sister-in-law who was hypothyroid and/or had thyroid cancer and how she felt like crap/looked like crap/had her hair fall out in clumps/got really fat/had bad skin and how it took about a year to get the situation sorted, but after they got the dose of thyroid meds right, she was great—perfect even.

These well-intentioned stories have started giving me nightmares. In my recurring dream, a woman who is a bit older than me tells me about how she had her thyroid removed and how she used to feel terrible, but now that she has found the right dose of medication, everything is normal and she is fine. This statement is comforting on its own, but the woman in my dream is clearly not fine: she has lost her hair, is thirty to forty pounds overweight, and has multiple chins and crepey-looking skin. Maybe the woman in my dream is supposed to be future me? I don't know, but I am scared that this is my future sans thyroid. I know I am being dramatic, and I should feel lucky that I am reasonably healthy, but I can't help thinking about how much I don't want to go bald and get fat. I am hoping that my endocrinologist can assist with my appearance maintenance so I can be energetic, happy, thin, have good hair and skin and stay cancer-free. Is that too much to ask?

I tell my endocrinologist about the plan to go ahead with radioactive iodine ablation. He is all for it and is quite adamant that it is the right thing to do. The surgeon was not keen; the radiation oncologist said it was up to me, and the endocrinologist insisted upon it. I am Goldilocks and the Three Specialists.

Everything is all set for me to start the last leg of my treatment. I am signed up for more waiting. More dates punctuate my future plans: in three weeks I switch to Cytomel, the short-acting thyroid medication that I will be on for three weeks. Then I have to stop all thyroid medication for two weeks. One week before I take the radioactive iodine, I have to switch to a low-iodine diet. By all accounts, I will feel like shit. After that, I will go to the hospital to take my magic radioactive iodine pill and then I will head home, where I will have to be isolated for seven days.

Time keeps flying as I reach for each date to pass and for an endpoint. I am relieved and looking forward to having it all behind me. I have had to be the patient, doctor, and advocate all in one. I am exhausted. This is partly because I am now off my regular thyroid medication and taking the Cytomel, which is supposed to help me not to feel too awful. Great theory, but I feel awful anyway. For my first week on the Cytomel, I was so tired and emotional I had no idea how I was going to cope. I was convinced that the dose I was on was too infrequent. I also felt a bit manic as I rode the ups and downs of this short-acting pill. Normally, your thyroid hormone is supposed to be fairly constant, without big fluctuations throughout the day.

I tried to talk to my GP about it. He wanted no part of adjusting this medication, since he had never prescribed Cytomel. I called the radiation oncologist and talked to the nurse. I asked her if they could adjust the dose because I felt pretty rough on my current dose. She said that they wouldn't adjust the prescription without me coming in for blood work first. But by the time I would be able to orchestrate getting blood taken and the results back, it would almost be time to go off this medication anyway. I told her that I was still working and travelling and I didn't think that I could get through everything I needed to do when I was feeling this crappy. She replied cheerfully, "Well, hopefully you can." That's it? That is all you've got for me?

Somehow I can and I do. I move through this phase and now it is time to go hypo for real. I go off all thyroid medication. I am a sloth. Thyroid hormone sets your metabolic rate. Without it, your metabolism and everything you do slows down.

Here is a list of the clinical effects of going hypo, from the information sent to me by Thyroid Cancer Canada:

- Tiredness, loss of energy, weakness

- Trouble sleeping, nightmares, or excess sleep

- Puffiness, especially in the face, and bloating

- Loss of ability to concentrate, memory loss, absent-mindedness

- Weight gain

- Anxiety, panic attacks, irritability, mood swings

- Depression

- Dry eyes, skin, and hair

- Hair loss

- Changes in menstrual cycle

- Joint pains and stiffness, muscle cramps

- Intolerance to cold

- Constipation

- Tingling or numbness in fingers or toes

- Itchiness

- Ringing in ears

- Slight changes in eyesight

I would say that I am experiencing most of these symptoms, but none to a severe degree. I am really tired and, paradoxically, I have insomnia. I am very absent-minded and am losing stuff all the time. I'm a bit moody. I feel sad a lot. If it is possible, I am even more intolerant of cold than usual, and I am having joint pains and muscle cramps, especially at night. But overall, I think I am doing okay, all things considered. The biggest trick is not trying to do anything. If I stay put, I feel fine. If I try to do too much, I get tired.

I am off work now, but it is not like a holiday, because I don't usually sit still on holidays. I catch people saying things like "Enjoy your time off!" and "Have fun!" It is one of life's injustices; when you have extended time off, it is probably because you are unemployed, sick, injured, having a mental breakdown, or you just had a baby. It is rare that we have the freedom or allow ourselves to take an extended leave from our work or our busy lives to do something that we have always wanted to do: to travel, take a course, pursue a hobby, follow a crazy dream, or get into shape. We live to work. If we are lucky, we like our jobs, but most jobs are rigid and don't allow for extended breaks. We are not free. If we did take a break, our colleagues would think we were nuts and/or lacked drive and commitment. We probably couldn't do it anyway because it would be financially impossible—we have mortgaged ourselves up to here with crap we don't want, need, or have time to enjoy.

I pressure myself to make the most of this time off. Then I beat myself up for not reading all the books I should read. I also thought I should try to learn a language or get back to my guitar hobby that has not been progressing well because I have just been so busy for the past, oh, twenty years. I thought I should watch some classic movies, because it would be cool to tell people I did that during my time off and I would be culturally richer for it. I watched *Breakfast at Tiffany's*. What is all the fuss about? Audrey Hepburn was horrible to that cat. I cross watching classic movies off the list of things to do. I know I should not squander this time, but I squander it anyway. If I had the energy to do all the things I wanted to do when I was off, I would already be back at work.

I begin my low-iodine diet to get ready for the radioactive iodine treatment. I am a lacto-ovo pescetarian—meaning

that I am a bad vegetarian and that I don't eat land creatures, but I do eat eggs, dairy, and all forms of sea life.
But, coincidentally, the low-iodine diet restricts eggs,
dairy, and all forms of sea life. It also restricts pasta, soy
products, iodinized salt and, by default, most packaged
and restaurant foods. This has cut out everything that I
eat on a regular basis. It is my low-food diet. It leaves me
with rice, unbuttered, unsalted popcorn, unsalted nuts,
unsalted peanut butter, fruit, and vegetables. I feel like
an anorexic supermodel, or like I have just ordered the
tasteless "special" vegetarian meal on an airplane. The
low-iodine diet, with its severe restrictions on my already
restricted diet, along with my innate and cultivated inability to cook and my overwhelming fear that I will gain
weight while going hypo, have led me to the only reasonable course of action I can take on the low-iodine diet: I
don't eat. Considering all of the above, I am pretty positive that despite my fears, I will not gain weight during my
stint going hypo. I now suspect that this would be physio-
logically impossible on the low-iodine diet, and besides, I
feel so crappy that I don't want to eat anyway.

For the entire time I have been seeing doctors for my
thyroid, I have been weighed at every appointment and, for
the record, I have weighed the same each time. That does
not stop the running commentary about my weight that I
have endured since I was diagnosed. Actually, this open
forum on my weight has gone on for much longer than
that. It is the curse of being a skinny girl. It is not from
my friends; it is the acquaintances, particularly female
colleagues, who seem to be very intrigued by my weight
chart and ass size. Apparently my weight and my body are

fascinating. I get so many comments and questions about it: "Are you gaining weight because of going hypo? Losing weight because of the cancer? Are you hyperthyroid from the tumour and losing weight?" I know that I think about it a lot, but I don't really want to talk about my weight.

However, while we are on the subject, the tasteless low-iodine diet would make a great celebrity diet. Maybe I should develop a business plan while I'm off work. It is a surefire way to shed pounds. All this intense worry, insomnia, and sadness about having cancer are also great appetitie suppressants! Dieters may be lucky enough to get stress colitis and diarrhea during the whole thing, too! It's almost as good as smoking! It's all great news for my waistline.

In stark contrast, men who know that I am going hypo, or that my thyroid levels are generally screwed up, never ask how it has affected my weight but will quietly, cautiously, and purposefully ask about its impact on my libido. Summing up, I would say that cancer is a great weight loss strategy but not so great for your sex drive. I am not sure if it is that I am profoundly hypothyroid or if I am just preoccupied with the whole having cancer thing, but as it turns out, thyroid cancer is not a great aphrodesiac. All of your thyroid cancer questions are answered right here.

The physical effects of cancer can take their toll and become emotional effects. So far, I have been lucky that my appearance has not changed, as it does for some people undergoing cancer treatment, especially those having chemotherapy. When I see people who know I have thyroid cancer, they say, "You look great!" which really means, "You don't look like you are dying" or "You look much better than I expected you would." If you look like yourself, it throws people off. Cancer is not supposed to be pretty. It can be cute, in the hopeful eyes of a bald poster child, or courageous, in the classic headscarf of a breast cancer warrior princess. But not classically pretty.

My friend's sister Beth tried everything to manage the effects of her hair loss through her breast cancer chemotherapy treatment: she found wigs uncomfortable, she thought hats looked strange at work, and she was really bad at choosing and tying headscarves. Finally, she just gave up on the whole thing and started going to work the way she was: bald. It works for men undergoing chemo and for men with male-pattern hair loss, so why can't it work for women undergoing chemotherapy? It is a relief to everyone when balding men finally let go of their youth and the comb-over that is ineffectively masking their receding hairline. We all agree that men look better: Can't we agree that sometimes women look better bald, too? And that they shouldn't have to hide behind a wig? I totally support this movement.

But some people get uneasy when there is too much cancer showing. It's too in-their-face. Beth's co-workers complained to her and their boss that her baldness made them uncomfortable. *I'm sorry, is my cancer making you uncomfortable? Let me put on this itchy wig so you don't have to think about it. This must be really hard for you.* The hat, headscarf, or wig and the accompanying painted-on eyebrows and pallor are fine, but bald? Bald is too much. It's too naked.

So not only do we have to live with cancer, we have to stress about making our workplace cancer-free, or pretend that it is, so that everyone feels comfortable. You need to expose just the right amount of cancer. You can't win. If you come back from sick leave with all of your hair, thin, tanned, rested, or—God forbid—happy, that is too much positivity for any of your co-workers to endure, especially if they covered for you while you were on your cancer holiday. Showing up bald, right in the middle of your chemo? That is just too much honesty for any workplace to bear.

After I heard Beth's story, I stopped trying to cover my neck scar. I used to obsess about buying jewellery to cover it up, which was not an easy task because the scar sits at an awkward part of the neck. It's too low for a choker and too high for a short necklace. I bought scarf after scarf, even wearing them all through the summer, except on the hottest days. I added both scar and dark-undereye-circle cover-up to my morning ritual. Now I just leave it. Some people try to tell me that they don't really notice my scar at all while they stare directly at it, unable to avert their eyes. I have accepted it, but I wish it wasn't there. A permanent blemish on my once-perfect neck, like the permanent blemish on my once-perfect health. But it's part of me now. Anyway, I figure it makes me look like quite the badass.

I CAN'T GET THE stupid *Spider-Man* theme song out of my head, despite its terrible tune and weak lyrics: "Is she tough? Listen, Bud, she's got radioactive blood." *Spider-Man* has led to the unscientific, widespread subconscious belief that contact with radioactivity may result in superpowers. I wish this were true. I have radioactive blood right now and have yet to see any evidence of a superpower, but

I did have a mug explode suspiciously while I was making a cup of tea and I have had two unusually good games of iPhone Scrabble, so maybe there is some truth to this theory.

I have taken a jagged little radioactive pill. It was a lot of foreplay to lead up to a fairly anticlimactic moment. I went into the nuclear medicine department at the hospital in Toronto where I had my second surgery, and they were extremely nice this time. One of the technicians who checked me in asked if I have thyroid cancer. When I told him I did, he said enthusiastically, "Well, not for long!" He obviously thinks that the fact that this pill can cure thyroid cancer is a medical marvel, no matter how many times he administers it. He's right, of course, it is an amazing treatment. I'm thankful that he was there to remind me.

I am called into a room. Another technician goes over the recommendations for limiting the exposure of others to me while I'm in my radioactive state. I am also lucky that I can isolate myself at home. If I lived just a little farther from Toronto, or if my radiation oncologist were just a little stricter, they would have to keep me here. It would have taken even longer to get the treatment because I would have had to wait for an isolation room to become available, and I would have had to stay at the hospital for three days in complete isolation. I think they really do their best to make the experience as pleasant as they can, but the nurses have to limit their exposure to radioactive patients because they work with radioisotopes every day, so it would have been a very lonely three days. It will still be lonely at home, but at least it's home. It's jail versus house arrest.

My pill comes in a big lead container. After I receive the instructions and put on rubber gloves, the technician moves out of the room, leaving the door open so she can maintain a safe distance but still see me and talk me through the process. I take the lid off and see that there is a smaller lead container inside. It is all very *Alice in Wonderland*. I take out the smaller lead container and open the lid. There is yet another container inside. This time, it is a regular pill container. I am expecting a little note that says "Eat me." I take off the top of the pill container, tip the pill into my mouth without touching it, and wash it down with water. The technician tells me to remove the gloves. She grabs her Geiger counter to verify that I am now radioactive and that the pill is inside me. And now she doesn't mean to be rude, but would I please vacate the premises immediately.

I head off with a very dear friend who is not afraid of a little radioactivity. She is fierce. Like Tyra Banks fierce. She drives me home. The person who drives you home can't be the same person that you live with, to ensure that one person doesn't get too much exposure. I have two big fears on the trip home:

1. That we will get caught in rush-hour traffic and she will be stuck in the car with me for longer than the recommended one hour of exposure

2. That I will vomit en route. En route vomiting would create so many additional problems:

    a.   exposing my friend to radioactive puke

b. causing a radiation spill in the middle of
    rush-hour traffic

c. not getting my full dose of radioactive iodine

We head home. My friend is very short, so she has
the driver's seat pulled up as far as possible, and I am on
the passenger side of the back seat, tipped as far back as
I can be, and curled up in a ball so that my head, neck,
and bladder are as far away from her as possible. The
two important factors in minimizing radiation exposure
are decreasing time together and increasing the distance
between us. We do okay on both fronts and are impressed
with our ability to be so far apart in my Honda Element.
We are not perfect, though, and are definitely in the car
together for too long. Despite leaving Toronto at 3:06
p.m., we hit some serious traffic on the way home, but
my friend seems okay with it. Partly because she is just a
good friend, partly because she is very scientific and there
is not a lot of evidence that suggests this level of exposure
will cause any issues for her, and partly because she likes
to live on the edge a bit. I think she assumes that the raves
she attended in London in the nineties are probably more
likely to be detrimental to her health than our radioactive
road trip. It is all very *Thelma & Louise*, except that it is
only an hour and a half and we don't die at the end.

The first twenty-four hours are not too bad. At first,
it is novel to be radioactive. This is medical humour, but
the colloquial way to describe someone who has taken a
radioisotope is "hot." You can imagine the endless jokes
and texts that ensue: *I am the hottest girl you know. I*

am hot stuff! I am a hot mess! I am basically a superhot superhero! Coming down from this excitement, I am still hypothyroid, I feel a bit nauseous, and my throat is a bit sore, but I am happy to be home.

The isolation requirements stipulate that my husband has to move out for the first three days after my treatment. If we were living the dream in a massive suburban home with four bedrooms, five bathrooms, and outrageous square footage, we could both stay at home. However, we live downtown in a hundred-year-old, one-bathroom brick house, which was not built with modern conveniences such as closet space, enough outlets, and the ability to accommodate home isolation due to radioactivity. My husband visits a couple of times a day and stands ten feet away for quick chats; we walk the dog "together" with me trailing far behind, which I'm sure looks odd to anyone who sees us.

My dog and cat are allowed to stay with me. My dog Molly is fifteen. Although I would never want to harm her, and do keep my distance, I can't see any potential negative effects of a small amount of radiation on a dog of her age. There have been no studies that evaluate the effect of human radioactive iodine treatment on pets, but in principle, it is best to avoid any unnecessary exposure to radioactive sources.

The cat is a bit more challenging. Romeow is young and has his whole life ahead of him. If he ever gets some form of cancer, I will blame the radioactive iodine, so I really have to keep my distance from him. He is a big, lovely, cuddly tabby. I have always thought that he is a pretty smart cat, but he is hopeless when it comes to radiation physics. Despite my efforts to explain to him that intensity is inversely proportional to the distance squared ($I = 1/distance2$), he wants to get on my lap and sleep in bed with me. I kick him out of the bedroom. I notice that the more I push him away, the more he wants to be close. I always thought I had a good understanding of cat psychology, but I feel I have now cracked the cat (and possibly the dating) code: the more you ignore them and push them aside, the more they want you. Everything makes so much sense to me now. (Not that I am dating, but my friends are, and I will always have cats.) Maybe I do have superpowers. Since I started trying to keep my distance, my cat has made it his mission to be near me: he *must* be near me.

On day two, things take a turn for the worse when the effects of radioactive material passing through my entire GI tract become apparent. I am off the low-iodine diet now that I have been treated and can eat anything I want, but I don't want to eat anything. Without being too graphic, let's just say that the radioactive pill has wreaked havoc on the lining of my stomach and entire intestine on its way down, so this problem affects all aspects of my gastrointestinal tract. The side effects are quite miserable, but I am still happy to experience this in the comfort of my home and I know that it will pass (literally). I tuck in and lie by the fire, binge-watching TV episodes and movies, reading, and napping. Friends leave care packages on my front porch and run away. I try to stay hydrated and keep my spirits up with a few intermittent phone calls and Skype sessions with good friends whom I will allow to see me in this state.

On the fourth day, my husband is allowed back in the house. Separate rooms for seven days, but at least he can be at home. To prepare for his return, I have to decontaminate the bathroom and kitchen. No one else can do it, which is fine, but scrubbing a toilet bowl is not the most fun activity for someone who is extremely nauseous and tired. Extensive research has been done on radioactive iodine patients to determine what areas of the house become radioactive; this helps people know what needs to be cleaned and how it must be done after treatment. I was sent home from the hospital with a number of informative handouts that explained how to clean up my radioactive mess. There was a lot of focus on how to clean up urine because it is the main route of excretion for radioactive iodine.

This research confirms something that I have always suspected: men are disgusting. It is a scientifically proven fact. By following radioactive urine with a Geiger counter, studies have confirmed that men who stand when they pee make a big, radioactive mess all around the toilet. One of the recommendations based on this study is that men having radioactive iodine who refuse to sit when they pee need to put blotting paper, like newspaper, around the entire base of the toilet to allow easy cleanup. The information makes me pause. Gentlemen, if this is not enough evidence that sitting down is the right thing to do, then I don't know what is! Sit it down.

I was also provided with some very helpful information on how to clean the kitchen and manage utensils when you are radioactive, because radioactive iodine also concentrates in the saliva and sweat. It is stressful and I feel

I have a big responsibility to keep my husband safe. I do my best, but I know that I am not perfect. The recommendation is to wash your hands a lot because your hands become radioactive after you touch your face or eyes, or when your palms sweat. Does that mean the taps become contaminated every time I wash my hands? The whole thing would be a lot easier if the radioactivity glowed; then I would know when I was making a mistake and what I should clean. It would also look really cool. Kind of like when you order a gin and tonic in a bar with black lights, only it would be my tears, sweat, saliva, and pee that is glowing. Awesome.

I also received useful instructions on how to cook for others in your household while you are radioactive. For example, you should not reuse a tasting spoon when serving others, which you should not do anyway because it is gross. The instructions also advise that you avoid a lot of contact between your hands and the food when you are preparing baked goods—like, say, when you are kneading bread. I have to read that again. The verb *kneading* implies that you need to use your hands, which are likely emitting radioactivity. Keep in mind that people undergoing this treatment *for cancer* have been off their regular thyroid medication for five and a half weeks, and off all thyroid supplementation for two and a half weeks, so they are now both profoundly hypothyroid and likely experiencing some gastrointestinal side effects associated with ingesting a radioactive substance *for their cancer*. So remind me again why they are cooking and baking for the entire family? Why are they kneading and baking bread? Could the family possibly cook for them? Maybe they could just get takeout for three days? Or they could get bread from a bakery this week? Or a friend could help with the cooking? I am cooking nothing and eating nothing and I have no dependants except for a deaf old dog and a very amorous cat, so I am thankful for that, too.

Despite a few rough days of house arrest, I am feeling really happy that this is it: my last treatment. The odds are overwhelmingly in my favour that I am cured. I went back to the nuke-med department a week after ingesting the radioactive iodine for a nuclear scan. They used a gamma camera to see where the radioactive iodine had gone in my body. This department is a model of efficiency—I was in and out of there in about half an hour. Before I left, I asked my technician if I could take a look at my scan. She said I probably wouldn't have any idea what I was looking at, but she humoured me and let me peek. I knew exactly what I was looking at, and I liked what I saw. I was looking for that lymph node. The one that has been big since the beginning and has been driving me crazy. I didn't see it lit up with radioactivity, which I will take as good news until I am officially given my results. I find myself infected with the nuke-med technician's enthusiasm for the radioactive iodine treatment. It is a clever therapy with a huge benefit that more than outweighs the negative side effects. I might not have developed superpowers, but the work of countless doctors and researchers has given me the power to leap over cancer with a single pill, and that is nothing short of heroic. I can't get my new theme song out of my head: "To her, life is a great big bang-up. Whenever there's a hang-up, you'll find the Thyroid Girl!"

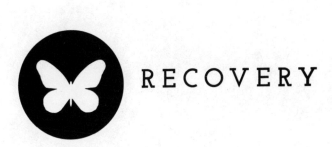

RECOVERY

I HAVE FINISHED ALL of my treatments for thyroid cancer and I am, by all accounts, cancer-free. The odds were always on my side, so I don't feel as if I beat them, but I feel good. Since the radioactive iodine, I have met with my surgeon and radiation oncologist again. They both said my lymph nodes were clear on the post-radioactive iodine scan and that I am good to go until I have a recheck ultrasound, scan, and blood tests in six months. Cancer-free: free from cancer cells. Yes, for now, and likely forever. Free from having had cancer? Probably never, or at least I hope not. Hopefully, I can retain the wisdom and freedom that being a survivor brings.

The late Hugo Chávez, upon hearing the shocking news that President Cristina Fernández de Kirchner of Argentina may have thyroid cancer, mused over the unusually high number of Latin American leaders who have been diagnosed with cancer. He said he was just thinking aloud (to the world press) rather than making rash accusations, but wouldn't it be interesting if the Americans had the technology to afflict these leaders with cancer and this was a U.S. conspiracy plot to remove them? The U.S. State Department described Mr. Chávez's comments as horrific and reprehensible. There were also more than a couple of holes in this theory. I don't think that an evil mastermind with the power to inflict cancer on someone would pick a cancer with a high cure rate like thyroid cancer. It seems like a lot of effort to not kill your enemy.

I never thought I would have anything in common with Hugo Chávez or President Kirchner, but now we are all survivors. I am cancer-free and Ms. Kirchner is, too. She just had to get through the hard parts first—and it is hard, even if you are the president and Chávez has your back. In the end, after all of Chávez's allegations, Ms. Kirchner's press conferences, and the candlelight vigils held by her supporters, she didn't have thyroid cancer after all. It was just benign thyroid disease. What a relief! Chávez was not so lucky. He succumbed to his disease after a two-year fight with cancer. His staunch supporters, known as Chavistas, still maintain that the American government gave him cancer. Everyone needs something to blame for cancer.

I will always need regular checks to get my thyroid levels sorted (they are still not right, but I am homing in on normal), and also checks for the unlikely possibility of recurrence. For me, cancer will not be a dark shadow, like it is for some survivors with more aggressive cancers. If it recurs, I will be almost as shocked as I was the first time around. The one element that I won't find shocking is the concept of my own death. We don't consider death very often, but contemplating your mortality brings a certain level of freedom. Appreciating life for what it is—brief and precious—is cancer freedom. We are constantly trying to forget that we are all going to die. What if we stopped protecting ourselves from death? It doesn't need to be so morbid. It might help us to focus on the things that are important and bring us happiness.

What would you change in your life if you were going to die in a few days? Weeks? Months? Or years? Well, the truth is, you are. How few days, weeks, or years of life does it take before you start living the life you want to live? Wouldn't it be better to live a shorter life with happy purpose and freedom than an unexceptional life of faux-immortality?

We also try very hard to forget that our pets are going to die one day, too. We get a puppy or a kitten and we know on one level that they will go before us in most cases. We know the projected lifespan of our cat or particular dog breed, but their death always seems very far away. In consultations with clients, these figures are checked and rechecked when going over the economics of veterinary cancer treatment. The numbers are somewhat artificial, because we are able to treat more illnesses in animals in increasingly aggressive and sophisticated ways. We can cheat death more than ever before. So, when clients ask me if it is a worthwhile investment to treat their eleven-year-old dog with cancer when the average lifespan for the breed is only twelve years, I have a hard time answering that question. All I know for sure is that without treatment, this dog won't make it past eleven.

There is, however, a point in animals and humans when the factory-original parts wear out and the body can go no further. And there are cancers that defy all of our treatments and knowledge. What we may know to be true on an intellectual level about our pet's or our own life-span is never internalized emotionally. When my clients are faced with the shock and disbelief that their pet has cancer, most of this shock and disbelief is focused on the fact that their pet is going to die, when really, they knew that from the start. We all knew. They always leave us. They always break our hearts.

A common request when clients are making these big decisions on their pets' behalf is for the cheapest, least invasive option with the maximum impact on the cancer—one that provides the best quality of life for the longest possible time. Unlike human doctors, I am able to provide a list of options, but the risk, expense, aggressiveness of treatment, morbidity, effectiveness of treatment, and anticipated survival times all move together along the same continuum. Some clients will opt for a moderate, palliative option—nothing too pricey or aggressive. We discuss it. Cure is not a goal, or an expectation. This plan should provide a fair to good quality of life for up to six months. They go with it. In six months, they are back. As predicted, so is the cancer, and things are no longer under control; nor can they be. But they are back for more options. Now what do we do? Now comes the hard part: you picked Door B. It's time to say goodbye. It's not fair or humane to keep going and I don't have a rabbit to pull out of my hat or any tricks up my sleeve. We talked about this day and about stopping. Sometimes, no matter what you do, there are no more options left. This is hard to believe when it is your dog.

As veterinarians, one of the options that we are able to provide is humane euthanasia. I believe this is the ultimate freedom—the freedom to die without pain. In humans, we resist when death is imminent, suffering is great, and there is no relief in sight. We hang on for dear life when life is no longer dear. We allow our loved ones to suffer. We watch them die. When a person wants to die with dignity, it becomes national or international news; a court battle usually ensues. When a high-profile euthanasia case is in the media, there are panels of bioethics experts, physicians, the terminally ill and their families. With all the controversy, I am always amazed that no one has ever turned to the opinions of doctors who regularly euthanize their patients when their prognosis is grave and they are suffering: veterinarians.

There are many reasons for euthanasia in my profession, but the most common are terminal illness and poor quality of life, with no hope of improvement or the potential for recovery. The outcome without action is clear: the patient will continue to suffer and then die. By choosing euthanasia, we can select the time and place. There can be ceremony to it. The family can control the situation and say goodbye. The patient does not die alone, and the death is painless. We are able to make this process peaceful, fast, and dignified for our patients. It is a ritual. We place a catheter in the dog's vein without the owner present, so that they don't have to see that part. Once it's in, the owner comes back to give their dog hugs and kisses and say their goodbyes: "I love you. You are such a good dog. It's okay.

You are not going to hurt any more. I love you so much."
Then we give an intravenous overdose of an anesthetic
agent. It is fast—shockingly fast. It always throws people
how we can move from life to death in a matter of seconds.
This is simultaneously the best and worst thing about the
whole process. How can you compare human euthanasia
to humane euthanasia in animals? Well, how can you not?
Death with dignity has definitely gone to the dogs.

I recently euthanized Molly at home. It was only six
months after I finished all of my treatments for thyroid
cancer. She was fifteen and a half years old and she was
just done. Not sick with any one problem, or at least not
one that I had discovered, just expiring, ready to go. She
didn't want to eat her favourite foods, go for walks, inter-
act, or enjoy life, not to mention that she was rather senile
and completely deaf. I put a catheter in her back leg while
she was on her bed in the living room. My husband was at
the front end, feeding her cheese (the only thing she would
eat) and scratching her ears. We were both crying as I gave
her the injection. It was fast and peaceful. None of us will
be lucky enough to have a death this good, eating cheese
in bed with your best friends in the world until the lights
fade out.

There have been moments throughout my life when I
wasn't able to reason through the death of a pet. For that
animal, at that time, in those circumstances, I couldn't do
it. I choked. This happened to me for the first time when
I was a teenager. I was working at the Humane Society,
gaining valuable pre-veterinary experience. I was helping
to euthanize animals by the dozens then, but my main
job was cleaning cages. After day one, I had pretty much

abandoned my lofty goals of playing with the animals and providing them with an enriched environment, training, and lots of love. I had also abandoned the notion that this might be a fun summer job. I lowered my goals to trying to prevent the animals from sitting in their own feces for too long and making sure that they had fresh food and water. We came in each morning to a chaotic mess of barking dogs; dog shit that had been paw-painted all over the cages; urine; wet, ripped newspaper; and scared, lonely dogs and cats. The puppies were the worst because they hadn't yet learned to urinate and defecate in one area of the cage. They were also the most active, and they would manage to get dog shit in unimaginable places: smeared on the walls and ceilings of their cages, in their dishes, and squished between the bars. The only thing you could do was get to work at one end and start cleaning. I would work tirelessly in one kennel room, only to see that the first row of cages I had cleaned was dirty as soon as I had finished the last. The work was never done.

My partner in these kennel-cleaning missions was a woman in her mid-forties: thin, androgynous, and bitchy. She had been worn down by the cruelty of people and was one of your typical animal workers who much preferred the company of animals to people and treated most people with disdain, myself included. She would stand over me while I cleaned the cages, insisting that I wasn't doing it right. Now it is true that I did not clean my shit the same way she cleaned her shit, but I cleaned my shit. My cages were spotless. You could eat off my polished stainless steel surfaces when I was finished. It was so frustrating to be covered in dog crap, urine, and sweat, cleaning my heart out, and then be told by this utter cow that my technique was all wrong. One day, instead of fighting her on it, I asked, "So, how long have you worked here?" I wanted to know what made her the leading authority on feces removal. "Seventeen years," she said. And it hit me: she had cleaned shitty cages for animals no one wanted for seventeen years. She had cared for them, fed them, loved them, and killed them for as long as I had been alive. With that in mind, I started to clean the cages her way. Not because I thought her way was better or that she was right, but because it was kind. I was there for only two months. Long after I was gone and had become a vet, she would still be there, cleaning the cages her way and trying her best to keep up with the never-ending shit and sadness.

While I was working there, I befriended a very gangly, unconventionally beautiful young dog with no hope of being adopted, because all she did was sit at the back of her cage trembling. It's a cruel world, where the beautiful extroverts always win. If you don't have looks and/or personality, you're dead. This dog was terrified by the whole Humane Society experience, thereby creating her own self-fulfilling prophecy of more bad things to come. Some dogs are too smart for their own good. She was great when you got her out for a walk, though. She was sweet, smart, and funny looking. I talked her up to my parents, who had more than enough pets. On the morning of her D-Day, my father said, "Whatever you do, do not come home with that dog!" as I left the house. He knew me well.

I got her out of her cage and took her down to the room where we put the animals down—the room where I would hold the dogs and cats for their lethal injections and then throw them into one of the huge bins full of wasted pet carcasses, their limbs and heads falling at unnatural and grotesque angles. We killed healthy puppies and kittens and threw them in the garbage. Why is it that the people who love animals the most, the ones who will be most hurt by it, always get stuck with this morbid task? It's so unfair. I walked her down the hall, put my hand on the door, and then turned around and walked her back to her cage. At the end of my shift, I took her home and called her Gilligan. We kept her for fifteeen years and she was a wonderful dog.

That was not the first (or last) dog that I dragged home for my parents. Their current dog is a gorgeous English setter who came into emergency during my surgery residency, with bilateral pelvic fractures and owners who did not want to pay for surgery, mostly because there was no guarantee that he would be a good hunting dog after a pelvic fracture repair. How can you put down a six-month-old puppy with a smashed pelvis who can't walk and is on no pain medication, but still wants to lick your face and tries to wag his broken tail? Answer: you can't. My parents fell in love with him over the Internet, and the newly christened Lord Byron found himself a new name and a new home.

When I worked as a veterinarian in general practice, I had a strict policy that I would not euthanize any animal unless I had spoken to the client myself. I needed to know why. One day, I came back from lunch and there was a dog in the back, waiting for me to euthanize him. I was being asked to go in the back and kill a healthy dog that I had never met—for no apparent reason—as an afternoon task. The animal health technician who had been manning the desk over the lunch hour and took him in did not even ask the owner why she had made this decision. She said the client was an older woman who was very emotional and upset. We were in Edmonton and her address was in a small town several hours away with only one veterinary clinic. I tried to call the owner but couldn't reach her (cell-phones were not common back then). I called the clinic in her town and they had no record of this dog. I went back to see him. He was a very nice young shepherd-collie mix who looked healthy. I choked again. I left him there over-night because I didn't know what else to do with him.

The next day, it occurred to me to check him for a microchip (microchips were not common back then either); he had one. I traced his name, owner, and address and they did not match the name and address of the woman who had dropped him off. The microchip-owners lived in Edmonton. So I called the guy and it turned out this was a really great dog, as I had suspected. His owners really loved him but the dog did not love living with the two small children who had become part of the family. Noth-ing had happened yet; he hadn't even growled at the kids, but this family had made a decision to find him a new home where he would be happier and where there would be no risk of negative child–dog or dog–child interaction. Fair enough.

Enter the guy's mother-in-law, who told the family that she had found a new home for their dog "on a farm" just outside the town where she lived. A farm! What dog wouldn't love to be on a farm? I think that depends on the farm, but no dog would prefer to be "on a farm" if "on a farm" is just a euphemism for death. The mother-in-law took the dog from his family and drove him straight to our clinic for a drop-off euthanasia before she headed for home. The owner came in and picked up his dog so that they could all regroup. Well, that's rather awkward, isn't it?

DEATH ISN'T ALWAYS SAD, and putting an animal down isn't always sad either. It's the why that matters. Sometimes it feels like the right thing to do and the best way to relieve suffering and find peace. But when it comes to our beloved pets, it can feel like an impossible decision. They rely on us to be their advocates in life and death. For a thirteen-year-old golden retriever named Kelly, that advocate was her owner and veterinarian, Greta. By all accounts, Kelly was a lovely dog, but it is always hard to know what a dog means to a family and what motivates them to pursue aggressive or extreme cancer treatment. Both Greta and her daughter were veterinarians. Her daughter had just graduated from the veterinary school where I was working as a veterinary surgical oncologist, and Greta was a practice owner and small animal veterinarian in our area.

Kelly had a long list of health problems, all of which were being managed by her mom. She had both ortho-pedic and neurological problems that made it hard for her to get around. Her mom was perceptive and noticed a change in her gait when Kelly developed osteosarcoma in her humerus bone. Amputation is the commonly recom-mended treatment for this disease, but Kelly was in the minority of dogs that would not do well on three legs.

Even if I thought that she would be okay on three legs, I would never push it with a veterinarian owner; Greta did not need to be educated about the wonders of three-legged dogs.

Osteosarcoma almost always spreads eventually, but Kelly's initial tests showed the cancer was affecting only her leg, which was good news. Greta would not amputate, but she wanted to do everything possible for Kelly, so she travelled to the States for stereotactic radiosurgery. This is the same procedure that Carney and Moses had; it involves a very sophisticated radiation unit that can administer a high dose of radiation to the bone tumour while sparing the surrounding normal tissues. Time, distance, and money aside, it is a great option, except for one problem. After treatment, the bone is weak because of the tumour and the radiation, which predisposes it to fracture.

Kelly and Greta came home from their radiation road trip and Kelly returned to our hospital for a course of chemotherapy. She was a star patient, always happy to see us, greeting her nurses and doctors with her wagging tail and smiling face. If you saw her in the waiting room, you would never know she had cancer. If you did know, you wouldn't have to ask if treating her was worth it. One look into her deep brown eyes would tell you. So would the way she constantly wiggled with enthusiasm or offered up her stuffed toy as a token of her gratitude. She was happy.

Just after Kelly finished chemotherapy, about four months after her diagnosis, she fractured her limb. Her owner and the leg were shattered. Greta still would not amputate the leg, but she did not want to euthanize Kelly either. She was an extreme client, and I wondered why.

Could it just be because she was a vet? As a group, we can be pretty extreme when it comes to our pets. Kelly was admitted to our hospital on emergency for pain relief and to give Greta time to decide what to do next. I talked to her about fracture repair as an alternative to amputation or euthanasia. It was not a great option, and there were a lot of reasons why this surgery might fail, but we could try.

Greta made the difficult decision to euthanize Kelly. When Greta got to our hospital to say goodbye to her best friend, Kelly was wagging her tail, smiling, and trying to use her broken leg. Kelly changed Greta's mind. She was not ready to go. Greta couldn't do it. She consented to fracture repair the next day. A few hours after surgery, Kelly was up and walking. As she walked, Kelly watched her newly repaired leg each time she put weight on it. Seeing and feeling that this limb was miraculously sturdy again, Kelly seemed genuinely pleased. It is unlikely that she understood much of what had happened in the past few months. Her leg had been painful with the tumour, then not painful after the radiation, then painful and non-functional with the fracture, and now it seemed to be working again, and she was comfortable. Canine cancer patients are blissfully ignorant of the anguish their owners are going through. Kelly was living in the moment and, at this moment, things were good. She went home with Greta the next day.

I received a lot of email updates from Greta after Kelly's fracture repair. Each one was filled with appreciation and good news about Kelly's life at home. The owner told me that we saved her best friend and that Kelly meant everything to her. She also told me why saving Kelly was so important, why she couldn't stop. I think she felt the need to explain her intense commitment to this dog. When Kelly was only six months old, she had saved Greta's life. She had accompanied her to the clinic to do a late-night check on a patient. Someone had broken into the hospital and, although you would not imagine a golden retriever puppy could be so tough, Kelly fiercely protected her mom and scared them off.

That alone would have been enough to make you want to do everything for your dog, but Kelly had done much more for Greta. In the past few years, Greta's husband had developed a gambling addiction and lost their entire life savings. He then became ill and bedridden, leaving Greta with crippling debt and the main caregiver to a husband who had put her in a devastating financial and emotional situation. Greta became clinically depressed and credits Kelly with getting her through that time. Her steady reassurance, smile, wagging tail, companionship, and unconditional love helped Greta to find her way out of the fog. Humans can betray us, no matter what they promise. When it comes to our canine partners, their only betrayal is that they will leave us before we are ready to say goodbye.

Despite a tough financial situation that I had been completely unaware of, Greta spent thousands of dollars and did everything she could for Kelly. She didn't bother asking anyone for their opinion because she knew the treatment was extreme and expensive, and she had already made up her mind. She just wanted her best friend in the world to be with her a bit longer. Kelly continued to have a great quality of life after her surgery and was using the leg well.

She was both pain-free and cancer-free.

The last email update I received from Greta came about three months after Kelly's fracture repair:

Subject: news about Kelly

Hi Sarah,

Last Wednesday my SUV was rear-ended. Kelly was belted securely in the back area, but she got tossed around. Her leg refractured and the pin was sticking out of the humerus by about 3 inches. We tried to come up with some solutions, but she ran out of miracles. My daughter, Kel's "real" owner, was fortunately able to visit with her. Sadly, my best friend is gone. She was euthanized on Sunday.

I never would have believed that she'd die for something so stupid, but she did. Just a few days ago, she was rolling around in the yard and enjoying the sunshine.

I just wanted to thank you again for saving her life and letting her be with me for a few months more. We really did cherish that time with her and she was truly doing so well. She really was happy until the end.

Warm regards,
Greta

I actually gasped when I read this email, I was so shocked. Sometimes, no matter how hard we try to stop it, death comes. I think about the person who rear-ended Greta. I wonder what caused them to look away from the road for long enough to hit Greta and Kelly. I wonder if they know that this moment of distraction resulted in the death of a brave and beautiful cancer survivor who had protected her owner more than once from the worst that human nature has to offer.

FOR ME, THERE IS nothing left to do now but go back to work. I have struggled with when I should return and how much work to do. At the university where I work there is a department called Occupational Health and Safety that I was supposed to inform about all this thyroid cancer business from the beginning. They determine when it is appropriate for me to go back to work and what accommodations the university could be legally obliged to make for me. I wasn't trying to go rogue, but none of this occurred to me until well after my first surgery, when I was told to make an appointment with the nurse in this department. The nurse who works there was not thrilled with my earlier unilateral decision to return to clinical work and on-call three weeks after my first surgery, without discussing this plan with her. She made it clear that this would not happen again. Now it's a process, and I have to break down what I do, and when I can go back to different parts of my job. It is a

mixed blessing to have a department like this. I have lost
control, but sometimes it's good to lose control, because
you can't always be the martyr that your work culture creates and expects.

I was required to go to see an Occupational Health and
Safety physician for an assessment before I could go back
to work after my second surgery, despite being in regular
contact with four other doctors. The doctor I had to see
had a severely receding hairline offset by a youthful ponytail. He was wearing cords and a flannel shirt. He didn't
really look like a doctor. We talked about my case and
about how my biggest concern was that I was not sure I
could be on-call, and that work on the clinic floor was
challenging because I was overtired from the treatments
and my low thyroid levels. Dr. Mullet Ponytail didn't
seem to know a lot about what a surgeon does, because
he suggested that I work half-days on clinics, which I said
would not be possible. He told me that the university was
required by law to comply with my back-to-work needs
and to modify my schedule as necessary. I tried to explain
to him that I am surgical oncologist; that some of the surgeries I do are hours long; that I can't just walk out the
door at noon with a half-resected tumour on the table; and
that I have to be there to take care of the patients after surgery, too. This is all-or-nothing kind of work and I didn't
think that a gradual return to clinics was going to happen.
My job is weird because, as well as being a clinician, I am
also an academic, so sometimes I just sit at my desk writing, and I think I can do that. I am doing that right now.
He scribbles my prescribed back-to-work plan on a form
and files it. On my way out, I tell the nurse that I would be

more comfortable with my own GP doing my assessment next time. My family doctor has been with me throughout this whole process and I think he is better positioned to understand my back-to-work needs. The nurse conceded, but I could tell it would be better for her if I would continue seeing Dr. Mullet Ponytail.

Four days before I went back to clinics, I attended a gala fundraiser for our Animal Cancer Centre. It was a big deal. Five hundred dollars a plate and almost four hundred guests. Brian Williams from CTV was the master of ceremonies and Jim Cuddy from Blue Rodeo performed after dinner. Canadian celebs! Rich, important people from Toronto also attended. Veterinary medicine doesn't usually get this kind of recognition—I have never used the words "veterinary medicine" and "gala" in the same sentence before. It was an amazing night. I was given the honour of speaking at the event. It was the first work-related task I had done in two months. It was an important night for me, personally and professionally.

It was time to trade in my velour loungewear, fuzzy slippers, and messy hair for a black backless pantsuit, heels, and mascara. It was time to bring it! Nobody knew that I'd had to cancel my morning meetings so I could stay in bed all day and rest up for the night, and that I was completely wiped out the day after the gala. All people knew was that I was away from work on medical leave one day, and at a fancy party the next, and that my picture was all over our Facebook page and the web site. I felt like I had to justify my big comeback to everyone I saw at work who had something to say about me, the gala, Jim Cuddy, and my black backless pantsuit. That's the tricky thing about thyroid cancer: you can look fine on the outside, but it takes all of your reserve energy to look that way. My energy levels, which used to seem like an endless resource, have limits now.

The next week I officially went back to work in the clinics, doing what I love to do: cutting out cancer and trying to make my patients comfortable and my clients happy. It is hard to describe how much I missed doing surgery. It is exhausting, though, because I don't have my stamina back yet. I love my clients but they demand a lot of my energy, and if I give up too much, I have nothing left for myself at the end of the day. In most ways, it is great to be back. It distracts me from navel-gazing about being a survivor.

Sometimes I completely forget that I had thyroid cancer because I'm so busy and everything is moving so fast and feels so normal. But then I find myself in surgery, removing a thyroid carcinoma from a dog's neck. It is hard to forget about your own thyroid cancer when you are performing surgery to remove thyroid cancer from one of your patients. I wonder how many people have had the opportunity to hold their own cancer in their hands—to ligate and cauterize its blood supply to kill it and render it harmless by dropping it into a jar of formalin, possibly curing the patient. Does it feel cathartic? Satisfying? Is it trippy? Absolutely. Mostly, I am struck by the privilege of knowledge and the trust that my clients and patients have in me. Every tumour I remove puts more time and space between me and my cancer. Every case I cut makes me feel more cancer-free.

Being back at work was great because I was doing what I love, but something wasn't right. My workplace had become toxic in my absence. I think that my workplace had cancer. People were so unhappy and everyone was always talking about how terrible the adminstration was and how much they wanted to leave. It's a major downer, but they did have a point. Things had changed. Most of my colleagues talked as if they were in a prison rather than at a university. It was as if they had no choice but to put up with all the crap and to talk about the crap endlessly. I wanted to say, "You can leave. What's stopping you?" But I knew it was fear: fear of making a mistake; fear of moving on to something worse; fear of moving generally. I didn't have this fear. My biggest fear is being unhappy and not doing everything that I can to change it and find happiness. Life is so short.

CANCER SURVIVORS WILL ALWAYS identify themselves as survivors and consider themselves members of this exclusive club—even if they have made it through the completely arbitrary five-year survival or remission mark. You are always a survivor until you are not. Ironically, the less aggressive your cancer is, the more likely you are to survive but the less you feel as though you have earned the right to call yourself a survivor. I am not sure how I fit in. Survivors get instant respect because they are perceived to have faced death but have fought and are winning. The reality is that most survivors cried, screamed, and had nightmares and insomnia; when that was done, they finally shrugged it off and realized that something was going to take them in the end. No one gets out of this world alive.

Thyroid cancer survivors in Canada even had their own name for a while. They called themselves Thyr-ivors. I can see why someone who is surviving and thriving and thinking about nothing but their thyroid cancer would come up with this name, and as one of those people, I find it clever, but it doesn't exactly roll off the tongue. Ultimately, the masses and Google were too slow to get the double triple entendre of Thyr-ivors (thriving, and surviving, with thyroid cancer) and they had to change the name of their organization back to Thyroid Cancer Canada.

Just when I am trying to figure out what do next, how to define myself as a thyroid cancer survivor and wondering who to talk to about it, I receive an e-newsletter from Thyroid Cancer Canada. I begin reading and notice information about a retreat for young adults with cancer in *Lake Louise*, and it is *free*! It sounds perfect and just what the doctor ordered. Having cancer is awesome. I click on the link to see how to sign up. I read more and it sounds just fantastic: young adults with cancer talking to other young adult cancer survivors about their cancer and surviving. They arrive strangers and leave friends. There are pictures of outdoorsy young adult cancer survivors smiling, hugging, and sitting around the campfire with the Canadian Rockies as a backdrop. It is so cancer-motional. I'm in! Except for one problem. Apparently, I am not a young adult cancer survivor. Young adults with cancer, at least for the purposes of the really cool free trip to Lake Louise with a group of cancer hipsters whom I will never become friends with now, are defined as twenty-five- to thirty-five-year-olds. I am, well, not. I don't qualify. I can't check that box. I am almost forty. I think I could pass for thirty-four, though. Maybe I should just lie about my age? I should start lying about my age soon anyway. Why not start with my new best cancer friends? If they think that I look older than thirty-four, I am sure they will just assume that my cancer ordeal has aged me prematurely, which totally happens.

I am not a young adult cancer survivor, but I am not an old adult cancer survivor either. I am in between. The old adult cancer survivors have their own self-imposed support groups called their friends, who are all getting cancer. I am a young/middle-aged adult with cancer. I feel like I did the weekend Steve and I visited my in-laws on their yearly bender in Destin, Florida. They are snowbirds who go to Florida every winter with their friends to golf, drink, shop, and sleep. Good times. Near the end of their stay, university spring-breakers show up with pretty much the same itinerary, except that screwing replaces golf as the principal activity. That's what happens when you get old.

Steve and I arrived during the retiree and spring-breaker overlap and didn't fit into either group. The university students had nothing to worry about because they were so clueless about what lies ahead. The retirees had nothing to worry about because they were done with worrying about what lies ahead. They're retired, the kids are gone, and they know that they will die, possibly soon. So everyone drinks like they are never going to die, or like they are going to die tomorrow, leaving all the troubles of the world on the shoulders of my husband and me. I need a nap.

AFTER I HAD FINISHED all my treatments and been back
at work for a few months, Steve and I decided we needed
a change and relocated to Florida. A new friend of mine
here, who is a Kiwi, and therefore extremely blunt and
doesn't pull any punches (which I like), asked me, "So,
why did you move here, did you totally crack up or something?" I guess it might look like that to someone who
doesn't know me. Only, it wasn't a cracking up. It was letting go and moving on. An amazing new job opportunity
presented itself at a time when my own work environment
was starting to feel a little toxic. I decided to go for it and
move south. I wish I had a more dramatic reason to change
jobs. It would make a much better chapter to say that I got
so pissed off about (insert random, tedious, paradoxically
low-stakes story about power and injustice in academia)
that I quit right on the spot. There is a certain appeal to
the spectacle of the Jerry Maguire exit to a job. Except
instead of taking a fish with me, à la Tom Cruise, I would
be waving a kitten around the hospital, yelling, "I'm going
to Florida! Who's coming with me?" The fact is, I looked
at the two jobs, made several useless pros-and-cons lists,
listened to my gut, and we finally agreed to just say, "Fuck
it" and try something new. We were up for an adventure.
I think that having thyroid cancer had a lot to do with it.

Now that I am meeting all these new people, I'm not
sure how to tell them I had cancer. I don't even know what
tense I should use: I have cancer? I had cancer? I have had
cancer? I did have cancer? "I have cancer" doesn't feel right
any more, which is pleasing. Should I bring it up at all?
Sometimes I try to work the "I'm a cancer survivor" thing
into a conversation, when it seems appropriate, but it's an

awkward segue. I am not sure how it will be received. I feel like I am bragging about being a marathon runner or wearing a Tough Mudder T-shirt. Other times I bring it up nonchalantly, like it is one of many fun facts about me that I share with new people, along with my best stories, which can now be recycled, retold, and embellished wildly because nobody knows me here.

Going through the process of making new friends is exciting and devastating in equal measure. Sometimes it's great. I never tire of hearing myself tell the story about the aggressive bull snake that was curled up in the bathroom sink and how I managed to single-handedly immobilize him by covering him with ice and waiting for him to go to sleep. The hilarity! It is anecdote gold. Sometimes it is hard meeting new people: there are so many stories that make up who I am, it doesn't seem like there is ever enough time to give my whole picture or to see theirs. But thyroid cancer is a part of me now, just like being a staunch Canadian will always be a part of me, and these fun facts and stories come out eventually.

Then there are the old friends and acquaintances, the ones I didn't reach out to when I first got the news about my cancer. I was so busy working, having cancer, and moving to Florida that now it is problematic trying to catch them up. "Things are good, had cancer last year, but I'm better now. How are things with you?" Maybe I could add this news to a vulgar Christmas letter, twisting tragedy into a happy tale that laid out on holiday paper and mailed or emailed to one hundred of my closest friends, many of whom I have not spoken to for one or two years. The annual holiday letter is the ultimate medium to euphemize death, divorce, cancer, and loser adult children. The holiday letter can be boring, long, self-indulgent, and impersonal, but one thing it can never be is negative. It is the Disney-fied fantasy version of yourself and your life. Every achievement is lauded as a roaring success, every picture is perfect. Any challenges that the year brought were met with triumph.

Finding the photos to accompany the update is particularly challenging for me. I am either the least photogenic person in the world or I am much uglier than I imagine myself to be. Some people are beautiful in real life but take bad pictures, like Margo Timmins from the Cowboy Junkies. (If you don't know who this is, you must google her immediately so we are on the same page.) Picture after picture of me is a true waking nightmare. I think the raw truth is that I am just better in real life. I can do a lot with accessories like cute shoes and my personality, and this can tip the scales toward pretty, but the camera screws it all up again, unless the lighting and all conditions are perfect. I dig up some pictures of myself that I am able to stare at for ten seconds without looking away and attach them to my cheesy Christmas letter:

Dear friend that I haven't talked to for years,

It has been a while since we talked, texted, emailed, Facebooked, tweeted, or Skyped, and another year has come and gone. I hope that you and yours are doing well this holiday season.

Things at our end are busy as ever! My career continues to keep me on the go, with international travel and speaking dates that take me to exotic places. *(I am exhausted from all of the travelling.)*

We still have no children, which means that I have lots of money to spend on travel, clothes, and my ever-growing shoe collection. *(Please don't judge me for not having children.)*

We also have tons of free time, and most weekends I have an afternoon nap with my cat, Romeow. *(See above, exhausted.)*

The other benefit of having no children is that I still have the body of my youth. *(That is to say, I still have the body of a ten-year-old boy, and gravity is kind to A cups.)*

Seriously, you should see me naked. I look just amazing and I often get mistaken for someone famous. *(Just the other day I was told again that I look like Janice the Muppet by a perfect stranger.)*

Actually, if you look at the photo montage below of the carefully selected pictures from the past year that show me looking great and living life to the fullest, there is a picture of me in a swimsuit to show you what I mean. No, it's not Photoshopped; that's really me. Merry Christmas to you. *(It's totally Photoshopped, with*

*chicken filet–style padding in the bikini top to give illu-
sion of actual breasts.)*

Despite all the fabulous shoes and still having naturally
blond hair at my age, the year has brought some challenges my way. I found a mass in my neck that turned out
to be thyroid cancer. *Quelle surprise!* Developing a surgical cancer as a veterinary surgical oncologist! Wowie!
What are the chances? *(I have to say this as an attempt
to pre-empt your telling me how ironic it is that I got
cancer. I can't handle hearing it one more time.)*

I have learned so many things about our Canadian health
care system and myself on this zany journey. I sailed
through my two surgeries like a champ and even managed to enjoy the solitude of isolation during the radioactive iodine treatment. *(I was a complete baby through
my surgeries and I cried alone as the radioactivity
ripped through my gastrointestinal tract.)*

Every day I kept thinking how lucky I am to have this
"good cancer," because it is curable in most cases.
Good cancer has been the best Christmas gift ever. *(I
have to say this or you're going to ask me if it's good
cancer.)*

Thyroid cancer is the fastest-growing cancer among
women my age. I am right on trend. Breast cancer is
so late nineties. Now it is all about the head and neck.
Generally, I am feeling really great. *(Not actually feeling
great at all.)*

Getting my thyroid levels balanced has been challenging. *(That is, it hasn't happened yet and it has been over a year.)*

I have found a new endocrinologist here in Florida to help me through it. She is a good listener and seems highly motivated to help me not feel exhausted all the time, which is very promising. Which reminds me, we moved to Florida. Why the change? Well, there were many reasons. Our new jobs are truly awesome. The university here is a wonderful place to work with excellent colleagues. *(I also find it so refreshing that I am no longer working with an utter sociopath. The only good thing about working with a sociopath is that they don't know they are a sociopath, so you can write about them in your book and they will have no idea that you are talking about them.)*

Getting cancer sure can help get things into perspective. Life is short, follow your happiness. *(And run like hell from your enemies; they just aren't worth it.)*

Wishing you and your family a wonderful, peaceful, cancer-free Christmas.

Love,
Sarah

I WAS REFERRED TO an endocrinologist in Florida to continue with my care. Someone needs to keep an eye on
things down here. Just before I moved south, I had one
more recheck. On ultrasound, some of the lymph nodes in
my neck were a little plump. The plan was to do a recheck
ultrasound in six months. My surgeon's assistant, Emily,
called me to tell me that she was setting up the referral
and that the new doctor's office needed to know my health
insurance provider and policy number. I didn't have the
answers to those questions yet because I hadn't started
my new job. She told me that she was faxing everything
down and someone would be in touch. She then washed
her hands of the project. Predictably, nothing happened.

As soon as I had an American health insurance provider, I called Emily in Canada, hoping that she could
help me get my appointment set up. She told me that she'd
already faxed everything. I asked her if she could call to
see about getting me an appointment. This was a big ask,
because from her perspective, faxing was as far as she
needed to go. I did manage to get the new endocrinologist's name and a weak promise that she would resend
the fax. In Canada, you have to be referred to a specialist,
and your doctor's office has to set everything up for you.
In the States, the system is a bit simpler: you pick up the
phone and book an appointment. I had no idea and was
still relying on Emily to make this appointment happen
for me.

I did an Internet search of the endocrinologist and
found that I was able to request an appointment through
the web site. Three days later, I received a call from the
endocrinologist's office to set up my appointment. It was

Friday, the fourteenth of the month. The receptionist asked me if I could make it in on the seventeenth. I assumed she was talking about the following month, because she could not possibly mean Monday. But no, she meant Monday, three days from now. As a Canadian, it is shocking to google your specialist, contact their office, and make an appointment for yourself without a referral, all within the span of a week. It probably could have been even faster if I had needed it to be—like if I had been panicking about a fast-growing mass that suddenly popped up in my thyroid gland, for example. I asked her if she had received the fax from my surgeon in Canada. No such luck.

I tried to phone Emily again to ask if she could re-resend the fax. I got a machine that told me she was unavailable and that I could not leave a message. What is the point of an answering machine that tells you that nobody is there, that you can't leave a message, and to call back later? This is all implied by the fact that nobody has answered the phone. So I used the card that I had been saving. I emailed my surgeon in Toronto and asked if he could help me get my records sent to my new endocrinologist.

The email resulted in immediate action. On the morning of my appointment, I got a call from Emily to tell me that she was faxing my records over right away, which was a good thing because the appointment was in two hours. She still couldn't understand why they didn't have the previous two faxes, since she had the transmittal records to prove she had indeed faxed my records over—twice. I asked her if she could call them to see what the problem was. Maybe? Please? I brought what I had of my records along, just in case the fax didn't make it.

The fax didn't make it.

I checked in and waited for five minutes until I was called into the exam room. Ten minutes later, I met my new endocrinologist. I didn't even have time to dig into my waiting room activities. My new doctor is lovely. She was visibly disappointed that she hadn't had the chance to go over my records in advance, but happy to have what I'd cobbled together for her. I was visibly disappointed that she looked to be about eight months pregnant. In Canada, this would mean you'd need to work with a new doctor during her one-year maternity leave, and you might have trouble finding one. I wondered why she would take on a new patient, given her condition. But we are not in Canada. She told me that we would get things started and she would be off on maternity leave for only twelve weeks, possibly less, and that she would still be checking on my results from her mat leave. Toto, we are not in Canada any more. Twelve weeks is nothing in thyroid time.

She spent a long time getting my history and then made a plan with me to work on my concerns. My energy level was still a bit low, so she wanted to recheck my thyroid levels and adjust the dose. I told her about the worrisome slightly plump lymph node that was hanging out in my neck and had been slightly bigger when it was checked six months ago. She wanted to do a neck ultrasound and a TSH stimulation test to check my thyroglobulin levels. If they were negative, it was unlikely that this was anything to worry about. However, if I was still worried, she would send me for lymph node removal and histopathology to be sure. I had no idea if that was what I wanted, but I felt empowered by the options.

I had my blood work and the ultrasound done within the week and my new doctor's assistant called me to go over the results. My thyroid had come in a bit low so we increased my dose. Hurrah! My unstimulated thyroglobulin was undetectable, which was really great news, but we would still check it again after stimulation. Hurrah again! My neck ultrasound showed slightly plump nodes, just like six months ago, which was probably insignificant but needed to be watched with another ultrasound in six months. We planned to set up a TSH stimulation test for the next month. She asked me what times would be most convenient to have this done. I was in awe. The TSH stimulation test involves using Thyrogen to see if you can stimulate any remaining thyroid cancer cells to produce thyroglobulin (if there are any). This is the same drug that I would have been on before the radioactive iodine instead of going hypo, if there had not been that pesky worldwide shortage at the time. There shouldn't be any thyroid cells left anywhere (normal or cancererous), so if any thyroglobulin is detected after TSH stimulation, you have a problem.

We delayed setting up the test, mostly because of my schedule and because I was trying to figure out if my insurance would cover it or not. I knew from previous research that Thyrogen is pricey. I couldn't get a straight anwer out of anyone about whether or not it would be covered. It definitely wasn't helpful that I didn't understand the whole HMO, PPO, co-pay lingo of the American system. I called the doctor's office and they told me to call my insurance company. I called the insurance company and they told me to get the billing code from my doctor's office. I called the doctor's office and they told me that they didn't have a billing code, and they couldn't seem to figure out if this was considered a procedure, a drug, or a test. The most I could get out of anyone was that they thought it would probably be okay.

The receptionist from my doctor's office who called me to set up the tests also asked if I could get my records faxed down for them (she didn't seem overly keen to call my doctor's office herself). I called Canada again. Emily was exasperated, but she didn't seem willing to try any method of communication other than fax, even after three (alleged) fax fails. I asked her if she could call the doctor's office in Florida, but she was not eager to do that either. I then asked if she could scan my records and email them to me, but she said she didn't know how. She might be able to get someone to show her, but she wasn't sure about that. She finally decided to photocopy my records and send them to me by post. Snail mail from Toronto to Florida. During the Christmas holidays. Perfect. Two weeks later they arrived. I scanned them and sent them over to my endocrinologist. Mission accomplished.

Immediately after my first appointment, I received an email survey from my new doctor's office. It contained some shocking, absurd questions and statements:

> We value our patients and their opinions. We are always looking for ways to improve the patient experience. This survey will only take a few moments but it will give you the opportunity to tell us how we are doing.

Did you get a call within the time frame you expected? *No, it was much faster.*

The staff member who answered my call was friendly, courteous, helpful, and listened to me, met my expectations, and had the knowledge to answer my questions. *Yes, it is bewildering.*

Regarding scheduling: Did you receive an appointment within the time frame you desired? *No, it was faster and was equally bewildering.*

Why do they care so much? Why did my new doctor spend so much time with me? Why did everything move so fast? Cynics will say it is because American doctors get paid more per patient and per test. They also have to compete for business, so customer service matters. Or is it just that these doctors are paid more, so they have more time to spend per patient? I suspect it does all come down to time and money—some people are corrupt and will do extra tests to make more money and other people will just find a job where they can practise good medicine and the money will follow. So far, as much as it pains me to say it, the American system is working better for me. I suspect that if I had been in the States when I found the thyroid mass, my treatment wouldn't have turned into a nine-month ordeal. Everything would have been easier and faster. I know it is not perfect here. I work at a university and I have good insurance. Not everyone has access to this level of care. Millions of Americans have never had health insurance, which I still can't wrap my head around. Some of them are genuinely horrified that health care is being thrust upon them by their president. They don't want Obamacare. They have the right to die of terminal illnesses and to kill each other with their own weapons and they don't want the government to get involved.

Life is all about trade-offs. You can have polite, stand-offish Canadians or you can have rude yet paradoxically friendly and gregarious Americans. In the strip clubs in Florida, you can have full frontal nudity or you can have alcohol, but you can't have both. Neither the American nor the Canadian health care system is perfect and you can't have everything. You can have a fast, efficient, high-quality system for the wealthy and well-insured, and shocking conditions for the uninsured or poorly insured; or you can have free, slow, bad service and good medicine for one and all.

Having said that, I have it on fairly good authority (I know people who know rich people) that, although we choose to think we have a universal socialized, fair health care system in Canada, there is actually an underground upper-tier system that caters to the über-rich. They pay their doctors cash for one-stop, no-waiting service, and there is always a place for them at the front of the line. The media recently exposed a queue-jumping scandal involving private health care in Alberta. (I love that queue-jumping is scandalous in Canada.) Private health clubs exist whose members are primarily rich male executives. They pay $10,000 a year to belong to a "health club" and get spa services, yoga, nutritional counselling, acupuncture, free towels, and a fast pass to the front of the line for unclogging their coronary arteries and for colonoscopies to screen for colon cancer. They also get the first doses of HINI vaccine when panic about HINI erupts and there is not enough supply for everyone. These pseudofacts make me mental. They disturb my overdeveloped sense of justice. (My overdeveloped sense of justice always leads to disappointment.) This is not the way things are supposed to work in Canada. Canadians are supposed to wait in line patiently. You can't mess with the system; you can't buy something that is free. In Canada, insanely high taxes go toward an imperfect and overloaded but high-quality universal health care system that ensures the same crappy service for everyone. Rich Canadians, if you want to jump the queue, take your money south of the border or get back in line.

HAVING CANCER HAS MADE me more willing to take a risk, in case I could be happier, and less willing to just accept that this is as good as it gets. It's made me demand more happiness from my life. It's made me less patient with the status quo. It is hard to find perspective sometimes in our work and personal relationships. We expect that things will not be perfect, but how much imperfection do we accept before we try to make a change? People remind us of this constantly: relationships are work; work is not supposed to be fun (that's why they call it work); there are always a few assholes in every workplace; every job has stress. Yes. But does every job cause you to have panic attacks, insomnia, and diarrhea? These are questions you should ask yourself.

When do you start listening to yourself and just go with it? When do you stop being scared about making mistakes and just follow your gut? When do you have faith that it is going to be okay? Don't sweat the small stuff is great, but what about the big stuff? Thyroid cancer taught me not to sweat the big stuff either—that stuff will kill you as much as any cancer will. I am still figuring out whether or not I made the right decision to move south. I miss my friends and family so much. I miss Canada. I was a bit mad at Canada for being so slow to get on top of my thyroid cancer after all of those taxes I paid, but now I miss it. I do love my job and the sunshine down here. I guess you can't have it all.

On the cancer front, things are good. My stimulated thyroglobulin levels came back negative, meaning that I have no markers of thyroid cancer. The lymph nodes in my neck are still a bit big. I get an ultrasound every six months and sometimes they are a little bigger and sometimes they are the same (a little big), but they always look like normal, well-behaved lymph nodes and not like lymph nodes that are full of cancer. I have read all my ultrasound reports, which makes me feel simultaneously better and worse. My endocrinologist always says that she is not worried but that I can get a lymph node biopsy at some point to "exclude maligancy" if I want to. I try not to worry, but it is hard not to sometimes. My conscious mind is fixed on the 98 percent chance of cure, 98 percent of the time, but sometimes my subconscious dwells on the 2 percent.

I have to have faith that everything will turn out okay. If things don't work out, I have to have faith that there will be another treatment, or good pain medication, or just legally assisted suicide. I'm in the South now, where a lot of people live on faith. I just had some obligatory Florida waxing done by an esthetician who is a divorced single mother with no health insurance and a kid with chronic illness due to Lyme disease. She is very happy with how things are going for her, and she has faith that God is going to help her find a new career, and even send the perfect man her way. I think it must be comforting to let Jesus take the wheel sometimes. I envy the freedom a faith like that brings. It's like having a higher power and a really good personal assistant and a matchmaker all in one. No need to worry about a thing: God has it all under control.

I recently experienced my first veterinary prayer circle. I was talking to a very lovely family about their beloved dog, Sam. A husband and wife and their two adult children brought Sam to us and they were all in tears. Sam had a large abdominal mass. Even with a CT scan, it was a little difficult to tell where the mass was coming from, but it looked resectable. I talked to the owners, along with one of our residents, our fellow, and a veterinary student, so there were eight of us in the exam room. We made a plan to take Sam to surgery.

The owner started to ask me, "Dr. Boston, do you mind if we...," but I had already finished this sentence in my head with one of several possibilities: "see Sam before surgery"; "ask you another question"; "call our family vet for advice"; or "call another family member and put you on speaker phone?" I was ready for those questions. I was not ready for "Do you mind if we all pray for Sam?" Now, I'm fine with my clients praying amongst themselves. I have a lot of clients who tell me that they pray and I always figure it can't hurt, might help. But as the family shuffled into a half-circle and we filled in the other half, I realized that they wanted us to pray *together*. They wanted me to pray for Sam *with* them. I was having culture shock right there in America, but I rolled with it and we all bowed our heads. I might be embellishing, but I'm pretty sure we were holding hands. The husband led our prayer with his rolling Southern accent and evangelical tone: "Our Father, please help us to get Sam through his surgery today. Sam is one of your precious creatures and we know that you are with him and that you will protect and watch over him and help him to heal. Please be with these surgeons during Sam's surgery and bless their skilled hands as they take care of our Sam. Sam is a part of our family and we know that you are with him and all of us today. Thank you, Lord. Amen." Amen.

Although my first reaction to the suggestion of a prayer circle was a combination of nervous laughter and an overwhelming desire to run out of the room, it was actually very sweet. I loved having my hands blessed before surgery. I hope that my clients will do that more often. For me, it was simply positive energy heading out there into the universe, and a way for Sam's family to feel that they were doing everything they could for him and to stay calm. It was advocacy. (And, as it turned out, the mass was easily removable. We were in and out of surgery in about twenty-five minutes, and Sam is still doing great.) So, prayer circles: don't knock them until you've tried them.

My parents' dog, Lord Byron, the now elderly English setter I rescued when I was a surgery resident, was recently diagnosed with a splenic mass. Byron is thirteen and a half years old and has suffered from arthritis in his hips due to the pelvic fractures he sustained as a puppy. The last time I saw him he was having a hard time getting around, and I had several talks with my parents about deciding when it was going to be time to say goodbye. There was nothing acutely wrong with him at the time, which makes it much harder to make the call and decide which day will be your old friend's last. Then one day he collapsed and was diagnosed with a splenic mass. The mass was bleeding and he was severely anemic. He needed surgery to remove his spleen and, unfortunately, I was too far away to help. All I could do was talk to my parents and their family veterinarian over the phone and give advice.

I have spent the past ten years listening to my mother tell me that she wouldn't do cancer surgery on her own dog, and I always sense a slight lack of appreciation for what I do. This is not to say that my parents are not proud, but hearing "I would never do that if it was my dog" and "How much did that surgery cost? That is just crazy!" is a bit invalidating when it comes from your mom. Despite this, I know that when my mother is discussing my career at the off-leash park or with her family veterinarian or over bridge, I am the most gifted veterinary cancer surgeon in the world and the reigning expert on all creatures great and small.

I was sure the discovery of the mass would be the catalyst to put Byron down. They had been considering it anyway and now he was severely ill and probably had cancer; the only options were surgery or euthanasia. I told them that they had my support if they decided to stop. Sometimes pet owners need permission to stop, and stopping can sometimes be the best thing for everyone. I thought that maybe my parents were this type of client, and I was trying to let them off the hook. I was wrong. They didn't want to stop trying, proving once again that you can never really predict what decisions you will make for your dog until it is you making the decision for your dog. Against all odds and my advice, they pushed on. They wanted to give Byron a chance. They had faith.

They found the money and their veterinarian did surgery on Byron to take out his spleen. I worried that he wouldn't make it or that he would have metastatic disease everywhere and they would end up with a big bill and still lose him. I also worried that if it turned out to be a hemangiosarcoma, because that is what it looked like, Byron would die of metastatic disease soon and they would be left with the feeling that they had put him through too much and it wasn't worth it. Those are two of the worst things that a client can ever say to me. But somehow, Byron pulled through. He did great. He seems to have more energy than he has had in months and he is full of beans in the off-leash park. Barking and wagging his crooked tail, he seems happy to still be here. I think that the splenic mass must have been there for a while and it was hurting him, like Lulu, my intern's, big splenic mass. The mass came back on histopathology as a benign hematoma. Lord Byron and my parents haven't looked back. I am not sure what made them have faith in their old friend. I think they felt he had given them so much over the years that he deserved a chance. Byron's whole life has been about second chances and about faith.

NOW THAT MY THYROID cancer is just about a bit of cancer maintenance, it's time to get on with life and stop worrying. In celebration, I ran a half-marathon and got a puppy in the same two-week period. The half-marathon because it seemed like an appropriately clichéd post-cancer almost-forty thing to do (take that, cancer!), and the puppy because life without a dog is lonely.

Trying to find the right puppy was one of the most terrifying and confusing things I have ever done. I have never had to actively look for a pet. Usually they just find me. Every breed I considered came with a long list of heartbreaking potential medical conditions that I have seen played out in excruciating detail. I wanted to get a puppy from a shelter, but the shelters in Florida are full of pit bulls. I don't have a problem with pit bulls but the province of Ontario does, and I didn't want to deal with any hassle if I wanted to bring my dog back to Canada. I had a lot of false starts, including meeting a German shepherd breeder with nine adult shepherds and eight puppies living in her kitchen; discovering a shady "rescue" group for fighting breeds that charges $20 to look at their puppies, which are in shocking condition, and $400 (cash only) per puppy for the privilege of "rescuing" one of them; and, I am embarrassed to say, even losing my mind temporarily and deciding that a low-content wolf hybrid might be a good dog for me.

In my defence, I have had a few exceptional patients that were allegedly wolf hybrids. I thought that I wanted one, but then I went to look at the puppies and realized I could never feel good about the decision. The higher-content wolf breeding stock are stuck in their enclosures and will never be pets. They looked miserable. Even the low-content wolf hybrids can be aloof and are not eager to please the way a dog is, and they are escape artists. The

German shepherd (100 percent dog) that was on site to breed with the wolf hybrids was one of the most magnificent dogs I have ever met. He brought me to my senses. I am not sure why the breeder was trying to manipulate his genetics, and thinking she could do better by mixing in something wild and crazy. He was perfect.

One of the pleasures of having a dog is meeting other dog owners and talking about what kind of dog you have. I realized that I could never come clean and say that I had a wolf cross because it would always feel wrong, which would mean that I would be telling white lies every day to perfectly nice dog owners. Even little white lies to perfect strangers can slowly destroy your soul. It was a useful but pricey lesson, because I gave a deposit to the breeder before I went to look at the puppies. I did this so that I could have the pick of the litter (see above, temporary insanity). I saw the puppies and my gut told me the whole thing was a horrible mistake, but the breeder would not give the deposit back. She said that she was going through some hard times financially and would be keeping my $400 deposit even though all of the puppies had homes and sold for $1,800 each. Serves me right for going down that shady road.

I finally found Rumble at our local shelter. I was checking their web site after many failed attempts to see if any puppies were available, and there was a litter of Australian red heeler–cross pups that had just been posted online. I stopped overthinking it, drove to the shelter the next day and picked him out. His mom was a red heeler and he was about ten weeks old. Everything else was unknown: his father, how big he will be, and even what he will look like when he is done growing. Perfect. I realized that I couldn't control the situation and I just had to hope for the best. He was in a litter of seven puppies and his shelter name was Cinco. We changed it to Rumble.

It has been so long since I had a puppy. I've forgotten how much work they are and how much fun they are. Just looking at him makes me happy. If dogs live in the moment, puppies live in the seconds, and every second is joyful: now I am playing; now I am peeing; now I am chewing your arm; now I am sleeping; now I am eating; now I am terrorizing the cat; now I am running; now I am playing with a squeaky toy; now I am out for a walk; now I am eating your sock; now I am running away from you; now I am sleeping; now I am smiling. Without being taught to, Rumble smiles when he is really happy to see someone. He pulls back his lips and shows his teeth in a silly, toothy greeting. People who don't know him sometimes find this a bit disconcerting, but I have always wanted a dog that smiles like this. I feel like I have won the dog jackpot every time he grins at me. Rumble is always happy and he makes everyone around him happy. Despite the fact that I didn't do a lot of research on Australian heelers or even know what else he is mixed with, Rumble is the perfect dog for me. I am not sure if he started out perfect or if he is just becoming perfect because he is learning what we want, or if I just think he is perfect because I love him so much. It doesn't matter he fills my whole heart.

People always ask me what breed he is and I tell them he is a heeler cross. Then they tell me what they think he is crossed with and how big he is going to get. About half of the people tell me that he will be huge and say, "Look at his feet!" and about half of the people tell me that they don't think he is going to get very big and say, "Look at his feet." The next question is always if he was a rescue (because he is clearly a mutt) or where he came from. Because we are in the States, people are not very shy about expressing their strong opinions. There is always a very enthusiastic "Good for you!" that follows when they find out he is from a shelter. It is forceful, with extra emphasis on the *good* and *you,* implying that everyone should be as good as me and rescue dogs from shelters. I am not sure what would have happened to me if I had gone through with the wolf-hybrid madness and divulged this information in an off-leash park in Florida. I think that people would be just as free about sharing their thoughts on this controversial topic and might yell, throw a bucket of blood at me, or give me a lecture about what a stupid, terrible person I am. Then they would go and buy a bumper sticker that says "Wolf Hybrids Suck" and slap it on their car with the rest of their raging bumper stickers. Rumble confirms that he was the right choice for me every day, and as a bonus, he is a walking advertisement for the fact that I am a good person.

And so I am a survivor (of a curable cancer) and a rescuer (of an adorable puppy). Both *survivor* and *rescuer* are powerful terms. I need to qualify them both because I am humbled by them and I am not sure if I deserve them, but they serve to remind me that both Rumble and I are very lucky dogs.

ACKNOWLEDGEMENTS

I WOULD LIKE TO thank you, the reader, for reading this entire book and for even reading the acknowledgements. I usually do it when I really like a book and I hope that you liked this one.

I gratefully acknowledge Noah Richler for seeing the potential in my writing. I am sorry that I did not know who you were when I first met you, but I'm also glad because I would have been too intimidated to talk to you if I had realized that I was sitting beside real Canadian literati.

I am thankful for my mom/first editor (sorry about the swear words in the book); my brother Alex/first fan (who firmly believes that his sister is the best vet in the world and will not be told otherwise); my dad/first critic/great listener (who was always honest and fair about my writing); and Steve/first audience/rock/amazing husband (thanks for listening to me read this book before it was good or a book and for your love through the rough patches). I am thankful for my friends and family for their support and for believing that I could do this (you are all in here somewhere).

I am grateful to the doctors who cared for me. Sorry that you had to deal with me. I know that you all saved my life and that you did your best within the confines of our imperfect health care system. I would also like to thank my patients, who make my days fun and my work meaningful, and their owners for trusting me with their hearts. Thanks also to Thyroid Cancer Canada for being a rare source of real information and hope for me and for everyone diagnosed with thyroid cancer. (Now everyone, please check your neck!)

My last big thank-yous go to everyone at House of Anansi Press, all of whom make me feel like a ridiculously lucky dog. Thanks to Sarah McLachlan for taking a chance on a doggie doctor who wanted to write, and very special thanks to Meredith Dees, my amazing editor, for loving dogs and funny girls, for everything that you taught me, and for always gently asking me to tone it down. (I think I get it now.)

A portion of Dr. Boston's proceeds from this book will be donated to animal and human cancer research and education. The rest she will squander on shoes.

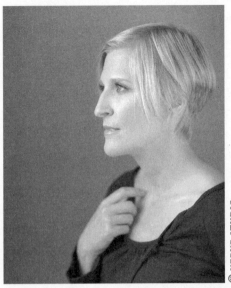

VERVE STUDIO ©

DR. SARAH BOSTON IS an Associate Professor of Surgical Oncology, Department of Small Animal Clinical Sciences, at the University of Florida. From age six, Boston knew she wanted to be a veterinarian. She received her Doctor of Veterinary Medicine from the University of Saskatchewan and her Doctor of Veterinary Science from the University of Guelph, where she did a residency in small animal surgery. Boston has practised veterinary medicine in various parts of Canada, the U.S., and New Zealand. She is currently President of the Veterinary Society of Surgical Oncology. Before her move to Florida, Boston was a faculty member at the University of Guelph. She lives in Gainesville, Florida, with her husband, Steve, who is a large animal veterinarian, and their dog, Rumble, and cat, Romeow. *Lucky Dog* is her first book.